GOOD FOOD, BETTER LIFE.

A Purposeful Guide for Health and Wellness

Martin E. Rollins & Joëlle Rabion

Good Food Better Life is a registered trademark.

http://goodfoodbetterlife.wordpress.com/

Good Food, Better Life: A Purposeful Guide for Health and Wellness

Copyright © 2010 by Martin E. Rollins and Joëlle Rabion

Designed by Kimberly Martin, Jera Publishing, LLC
Manufactured in the United States of America

10 9 8 7 6 5 4 3 2 1

The Library of Congress has catalogued this edition as follows:
Rollins, Martin and Rabion, Joelle
Good Food, Better Life:
Includes biographical references and index.
1. Self Help 2. Health. 3. Nutrition. I. Title.

ISBN: 144952561X
ISBN-13: 9781449525613

Dedicated
to those who seek to remove food as a distraction
on their way to a more inspirational life.

Acknowledgments

We would like to acknowledge Joshua Rosenthal for his inspiration to create the Institute for Integrative Nutrition (IIN), a school that is centrally focused on producing practitioners who learn to heal the whole person and not be concerned only with symptoms.

Before IIN, we personally had lost our way with food. We had become too political, philosophical and rigorous around eating and here we learned to heal ourselves first before serving as a mirror for others.

For Pat Lee, our editor, who accelerated and facilitated this book. For Virgie & Michael Rollins, Sr. and Polly Rabion for their steady support, also for tolerating our regular dietary experimentation.

To all our dear friends and clients who continue to bring us from theory to practice.

And finally to our practice of stillness via yoga, qi gong and other inspirational sources which ease the quietness that allows us to cultivate the love that we all are.

Contents

It is not about the food or the possible helplessness that surrounds it. It is about healing the source that allows for all great abundance to pour into every facet of our lives.

Preface

What are we all contributing in our own cultures that creates or perpetuates sickness in our loved ones? How much responsibility do we have in these relationships? We need to hold ourselves accountable.

Watching the New Orleans 2005 tragedy of Hurricane Katrina and its aftermath was a huge catalyst for us to seek training in holistic nutrition. While many concerned themselves with logistical, structural and emergency breakdowns, our focus was on the people and their years of nutritional inadequacy. It opened us up to a completely different type of discussion as we watched the situation unfold. While the press exploited the most sensationalist stories, I came to see that my hometown of Detroit could easily be in this same situation. I saw my family and extended family's issues with food and the deaths it brought. Joelle was aghast at the raw helplessness. Later, we each saw ourselves and what we easily attributed to our own struggles with food. This is where it begins: right in the heart of a neighborhood, right where your loved ones sleep, where you work. This is where the lights of the press should be shining.

We began to see how the collective mentality of a culture – whether at the office, at home or within a community – can have a positive or negative effect when it comes to food. In New Orleans, we witnessed the exposure of many of the people in the lower ninth ward who suffered from disabilities (i.e. missing their limbs, in wheelchairs due to a chronic illness such as diabetes). This prompted us to study with a greater focus on the family nucleus, on our communities, work cultures and our day-to-day interactions as the questions and answers to all of our disabilities. This, of course, wasn't something only we had discovered, and it didn't emerge as a "eureka" moment. It did, however, launch a methodical analysis that became the foundation for a road to personal happiness.

We know that people don't consciously want to do harm to themselves. We realize that our relationships to people, places and things have a way of putting us into a spiraling scenario either up towards success or down to despair. We are always heading into a direction whether we know it or not. Our relationships with our mother, father, siblings, friends, colleagues and lovers can drive us. What we saw in New Orleans was despair. The questions being asked were: was it FEMA's fault? George Bush's fault, or was it racial disparities or the Army Core of Engineers? Who knows? At this point, does that really matter? From our perspective the real question was: what was going on in their local culture where people were experiencing such profound depression, that they gave up control of their own bodies to the whims of the collective around them. This is the puzzle we held onto, have focused our practice on and what led to this book that you now hold.

Introduction

When it comes to the importance of eating quality foods, your diligence to do so does not matter - unless you are using it for purpose.

What do I mean when I say purpose?

Poor quality food is a distraction. You know the story by now: it leads to inflammation, which leads to chronic disease, which eventually leads to debilitation. It is a distraction that derails you from what you are supposed to be doing in your life.

You are here for a reason. To know this, to be engaged with purposefulness, there is a catch: you first have to own your experiences—all, *making no excuses for them*—to see what your life is telling you. If you do not like the present results then you must take charge of changing them.

We are not poor in spirit, we are not alone, and we are not unloved. We are love; and all of our experiences—regardless if they are negative or positive—serve us perfectly. The experiences we have are produced based on the ideas we have of ourselves, nothing more nothing less. The experiences that occur in our lives are not judgments, only reflections. We simply have to own them and know where we want to go before changes can be made.

You had that idea didn't you? You dreamed of being this person or that person for this or that reason. But your real purpose has something else in mind. It may have come to you intuitively, in daydreams, via certain events or another person's observations. Your life is calling to you, but you may be avoiding it because you are afraid. Perhaps the money is not enough, there is no celebrity in it, or nobody around you will support you.

This fear may cause most of us to have a problem with being alone with our own mind. Advertising companies understand this; for this reason, they put computer screens in elevators and at grocery store checkouts. We stay distracted and one distraction can be connected to everything else we think and do. Companies, family and friends tell you what to eat, who to spend time with and where to work. You find yourself in pieces. You are a pilot with no landing strip. This may be manifested in one area in your life, or all of them, causing you to take erratic steps using someone else's ideas.

Purpose begins when you start to recognize what is going on in your life. Not just the problems that you might have with your mate, your job, your parents or your finances. This begins when you own - take charge of - the experiences of the people, places and things around you. Many answers will be uncovered when you begin to take notice of your surroundings. You will begin to better understand your hobbies, your mate, friends and the importance of them in your life. You, perhaps, will also find your life's work, your "real career". You will come to know how it stems from the tools you were born with. It is about awareness, it is about you and your evolution into the full expression of yourself.

With this book we get you started on your purposeful path through food. The food you ingest can lead you to the truth. Once you develop the habit of eating quality food you begin to reduce a few of the obstacles – to *yourself*. You will begin to see that you need not be penetrated by friends and family who need your food misery to contribute to their own. Commercials for nutritionless foods become less distracting and more comical. Your body begins to heal, and with that you begin to think more clearly. New people gravitate to you, those who subscribe to your new manner of thinking. You begin to help those still suffering in your old way of thinking. Your path/purpose becomes more identified. Most importantly, you find that you are in charge of how you feel; you are shored up and now more in command of your life, along with being completely accountable for its results.

Life is, of course, not all about the food—whether you are eating poorly or what is considered the best food in the world—the question is still 'is the food or anything else distracting me into merely existing rather than living?' You are a loving being—whether you know it or not—and you are looking for the best opportunities to experience and know this for yourself. Let your new life of self-directed kindness with food from nature guide your path to purpose.

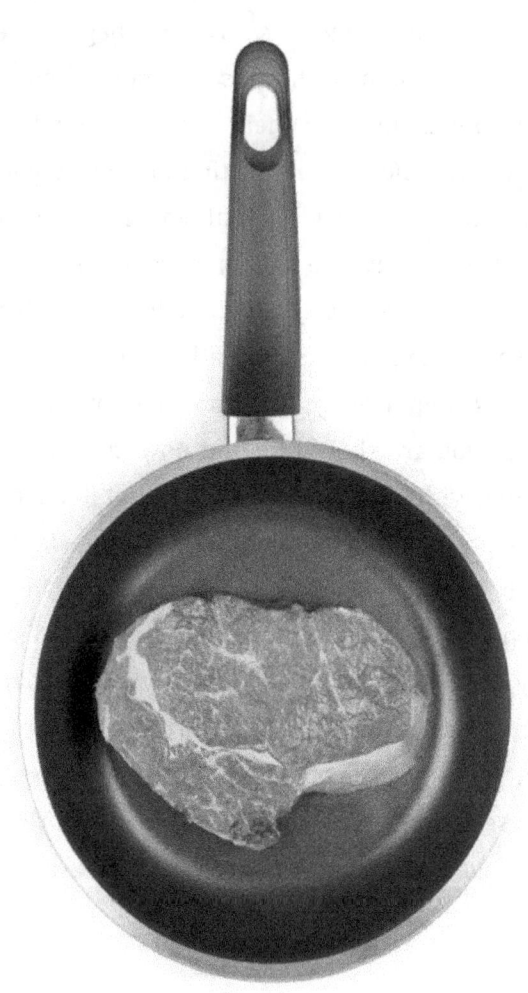

Protein

Palm-Sized Power

Eating animal protein can be debated as an ethical, philosophical, political, religious, moral or even a financial issue. But be aware that your body is not really concerned with opinions. Your body is instead looking for a physiological balance through the best answers to the questions: What is my blood type? What is my ancestry? What is the constitution of my parents?

Are you currently eating based on your origins? And are you paying attention to the possible fractures of that lineage? If you have a misunderstood heritage you will have to listen a little closer for which foods your body is asking for. For example, being African American means I have to understand a possibly more complex personal history with food. I ask: how much protein do I need? What type of protein works best for me?

These questions can be further challenged within a relationship. When I was married, my wife and I went from being meat-eaters to vegetarians to vegans. This process was based on her weight control and my own laziness towards cooking. What I learned was: from some meat to no meat was disastrous, for me. I am blood type O+, the oldest, "hunter-gatherer" blood type: my body operates best with animal protein. Fatigue, muscle loss and chest pains were common for me during this time. To combat this, I would further tout the vegan lifestyle, as though my suffering made me a better person than meat-eaters. It was political, it was philosophical and it was laziness that didn't serve my body well. My wife's blood type was AB which allows for more of a vegan lifestyle, a vegetable-agriculture way of eating. This doesn't mean she could avoid acknowledging her ancestry or parents' constitution. It just meant being vegan was more of a successful base for her, though she continues to seek what works best for her digestion.

What works for me might not work for you. There is a lot of trial and error involved. Get familiar with your history. Listen to your body. Don't get caught up in someone else's politics. Know that you are a meat-eater, vegetarian or vegan because your body is asking for this approach, not because of a philosophy. Your pancreas isn't voting in the next election. But if you let it and the rest of your body tell you what it needs, your decision-making will be better served.

PROTEIN: WHAT IS IT AND WHY DO I NEED IT?

As a former vegetarian (for 20 years) I learned that my body feels better when I provide it with some animal protein. My thoughts *seem to come quicker, I have sustained energy, I feel more ground-ed. Once you know your blood type, you'll have a good sense of whether your body will run best on proteins or carbohydrates. Start to explore and experiment: eat meals with and without animal protein and see how you feel right afterwards, an hour later and two hours later.*

Protein comes from the Greek 'prota', meaning "of primary importance." A necessary part of every cell in the human body, protein is crucial to our body's growth – muscles, bones, teeth, nails, hair – and minute-to-minute regulation and maintenance of vital functions: all tissues depend on it, blood can't clot without it. Protein provides the body with energy, is the building block of cells and tissues and the principal source of enzymes and hormones. Protein enables vitamins and minerals to perform properly in the body and assists in maintaining the acid-alkaline (pH) balance.

The basic units of protein are amino acids. Eight essential ("essential" because the body alone cannot produce them) amino acids are required to make a complete protein in the body. The liver produces 80% of the necessary amino acids; the remaining 20% must come from your diet. Provided you consume these eight essential amino acids each day, you meet your protein needs.

HOW MUCH PROTEIN DO I NEED?

Though our bodies are good at recycling protein, we use it constantly so it's important to replace. Protein needs depend on our size, age and activity levels; if you exercise vigorously your body will require more protein. If you need a guideline: to multiply your body weight by .37 for the amount of grams/day, or, roughly,

Women (145 lbs):	53 grams /day
Men (200 lbs):	74 grams/day

When eating animal protein, aim to keep the portion no larger than the palm of your hand. Vegetarians can double their protein portion. Too much animal protein contributes to acidity, obesity, osteoporosis, heart disease and cancer – not to overlook the negative environmental impact.

WHAT FOODS ARE BEST?[1]

Protein is found in meat, fish, dairy, eggs, legumes, nuts, seeds and grains. Scientifically, a protein is a protein whether it comes from animals or plants. However, each protein source affects our energy levels differently.

Learn your blood type. It can be useful in determining whether your body is more suited for animal or vegetable proteins. The digestive systems of people with blood type O can better absorb meat than other blood types. If you come from a meat-eating culture, it will make more sense for you to incorporate meat in your diet than if you are from a long lineage of vegetarians from India. Bolivians are largely a grain-eating culture; quinoa and legumes will provide adequate protein.

With animal protein, aim to purchase the highest quality possible. This means buying organic, naturally fed, cage-free or wild. Try for fresh before frozen. Conventional animal protein production has increasingly relied upon the use of hormones, antibiotics, and unnatural feed, as well as caging processes that allow for little or no mobility during the animal's life.

What	Why	How
Sardines	Complete protein source: eat the whole fish! Great source of calcium.	Supermarket provides many options, share with your cat!
Eggs	Complete protein source, whole food. Go for organic, nutrition-rich, free-run eggs. You will see and taste the difference in brighter yolk and flavor.	Any way you like them. (brown or white shells = the same content)
Yogurt	Complete protein source with A and D vitamins, many of B-complex. Probiotic attributes provide the bacteria needed for digestion and prevention of many gut disorders.	Only natural yogurt with live, active yogurt cultures, such as Greek or Fage brand yogurts. **not** flavored or "low-fat"
All grain and vegetable (non-meat) sources of protein	High protein content promotes physical growth and development without meat's cholesterol or saturated fat that can contribute to heart disease	See below for details
Quinoa: my favorite!	50% protein, high in iron and fiber	Boil in water, cooks up in 12 minutes! Delish and super versatile.
Brown rice, buckwheat (kasha or groats), oats	Good source of protein, fiber and manganese	Breakfast! Kasha has a unique flavor, taste, and see for yourself!
Rye, amaranth, wheat germ	Super high in protein, fiber and iron	Whole rye bread is a nice alternative

Sprouts	50% protein, high in vitamins, minerals, antioxidants, *Essential Fatty Acids (EFA), enzymes protect from toxic build up, strengthen immune response	Toss on a salad, in stir fry, scrambled eggs, brown rice, pasta, soup, mmmm!
Beans (legumes not green beans)	Contain a complete set of amino acids; excellent source of fiber, iron and folic acid. Great carbohydrate for diabetics or those with sugar imbalances as beans gradually increase blood sugar levels. Contain the phytochemical diosgenin, inhibits cancer cells from multiplying. Strengthen kidneys and adrenal glands	Your digestive system may require time to adjust to beans, to learn how to break them down in the intestines. Start by soaking them until the center is opaque when sliced open; soaking helps with gassiness, as does a teaspoon of vinegar. Or add an inch of seaweed, like kombu or kelp.
Mung beans, black beans, lentils	High in folate, iron and fiber, low in fat. Contain protein equal to beef	Easiest to digest. Boil, add tumeric for extra healing and flavor, delicious!
Garbanzo beans (chickpeas)	Amazing source of iron, protein, fiber	Eat cold in salads, make hummus: quick & easy!
Adzuki beans, black-eyed peas	Benefit kidneys: major iron and fiber	Drink the cooking water as tea! Add tamari and squash, mmm.
Seaweed, algae, spirulina	Complete proteins with all 22 amino acids, the entire vitamin B complex including B12, carotenes, minerals and EFAs	Eat wakame chilled as salad. Sprinkle smoked seaweed onto brown rice, eggs, in stir fry, add to smoothies.
Nuts: always raw	Good source of protein and essential fatty acids	Unroasted, unsalted. Not dry roasted. Raw. On salads, stir-frys, soups, snacks.

Seeds: hemp, pumpkin, chia	huge protein (25%) and EFAs, high in zinc. Huge Omega-3 content: pumpkin 15%, hemp 20%, chia 30%. Chia is loaded with nutrients and great for weight loss	Raw, in salads. Soak chia, use in gel form in smoothies and salads.
Edamame	Compares in quality to animal protein, rich in calcium, iron, zinc, B vitamins	Boil, lightly salt and eat: yum! This is good soy.
Tofu	Mineral-rich, compares in quality to animal protein, contains all 8 essential amino acid. Rich in calcium, iron, zinc, B vitamins. (We are not fans of soy, see *Vegetables* chapter.)	Cut into cubes, stir fry, or scramble, as with eggs. Use in place of sour cream, cheese, milk and cottage cheese. Adds richness, texture to any recipe; light, creamy character takes on any flavor, savory or sweet.

*Essential Fatty Acids (EFAs) are fatty acids that the body requires for good health which we must ingest as the body can't make them from other food components

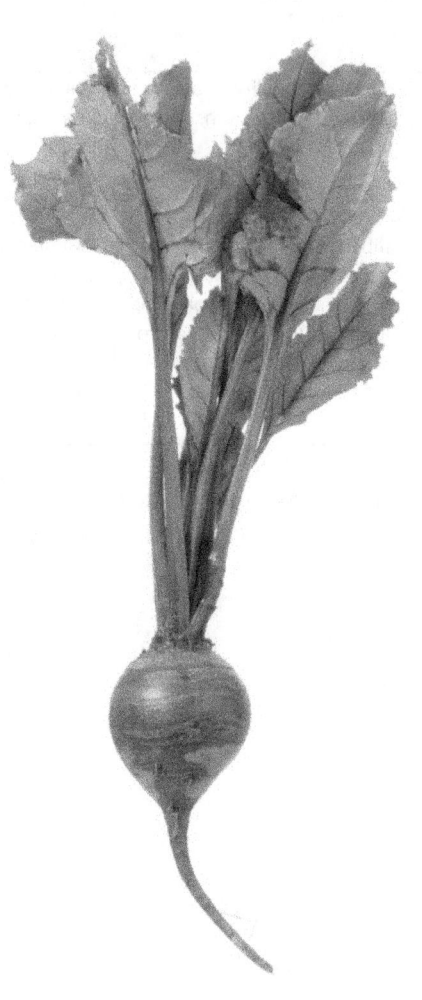

Vibrant Vegetables

V egetables, in many cases, take an outside force for us to learn to eat them. They may be introduced by a parent, mate or recommended by a doctor. Maybe because of the taste, texture and lack of advertising, we don't steam up a pot full while chanting, "This is good for my body, this is really good for my body." If we didn't have this outside force we might go our whole life not eating them. That life wouldn't be pretty for our body's functionality.

For people whose blood type is A, B or AB it becomes more important that you eat your vegetables. Theses blood types succeeded O+ as access to animal meat dwindled and people began to rely more on crops and vegetables. Grains and plants would eventually become staples for generations, thus changing the structure of blood for that ancestry.

Every culture eats vegetables in some form. I was raised with mustard and collard greens, cabbage, spinach and broccoli. But most of these greens were served with enough other food to properly crowd them out. We just want to remind you that vegetables can take precedence on your plate; they can be the entrée rather than just having them added to satisfy an onlooker. But the most important points to remember about vegetables are their variety and their extraordinary health benefits. Vegetables can alleviate or eliminate chronic disorders that you may be taking drugs to combat. Looking at them in this way can be eye-opening – let's take a look at their stories.

EAT YOUR VEGETABLES! ....WHY??[2]

Even if your genetics and lifestyle are working against you, your diet makes an enormous difference in your health and healing. Simply put, the more fruits and vegetables you eat, the more nutrition you get and the less your risk of illness and disease. In addition, these foods are most effective when attempting to reach your ideal weight.

Greens are, without humility, The Miracle Food.

Ounce for ounce they pack nearly 20 times more essential nutrients than any other food. Dark, leafy greens provide the greatest benefits of all the greens. The most therapeutic ingredient in green foods is chlorophyll, the "blood" of plants: it boosts the immune system, treats illness, detoxifies the liver, and calms the nerves. The darker the greens, the more fibrous and slightly bitter in taste. You can eat them raw, or cooking/steaming/blanching them lightly (just till they turn bright) will ease digestion. My preferred cooking method is briefly sautéing them in garlic and a high-quality olive oil.

What	Why	How
Dark leafy greens: kale, collards, Swiss chard	Excellent source of calcium, chlorophyll, iron, vitamins A, C, E, K. Potassium, phosphorous, zinc. Full of fiber, folic acid, micronutrients, phyto-chemicals. Great for omega-3 fatty acids	Steam or blanche, just until they turn bright green.
Leafy greens: beet greens, spinach, parsely, mizuna, also bok choy, napa/ red/green cabbage	High sources of vitamin A, chlorophyll, calcium, sodium, magnesium, iron. Effective for kidney and urinary difficulty	Steam, or lightly sautée in olive oil and garlic. Cabbage loses its bitterness when cooked.
Bitter Greens: mustard greens, arugula, dandelion greens, escarole, chicory and watercress	Known for their powerful ability to clean out toxins and fats from the body. Incorporate daily if interested in weight loss or in cleansing the body	Delicate structure, slightly lighter in color, strong, bitter, refreshing taste. Eat raw or prepared as above.
Green vegetables in general:	Purify the blood, their antioxidants help prevent cancer, boost immune system, promote healthy intestinal flora, improve liver, gall bladder, kidney function; lift the spirit, clear congestion in the lungs, reduce mucus, improve circulation, keep skin clear, facilitate weightloss. Folic acid prevents heart disease. Vitamin K in chlorophyll enhances adrenal activity	Unleash their healing power by eating them raw or lightly cooked.

MORE VEGETABLES

The healing power is unleashed if eaten raw or lightly cooked (½ cup cooked or 1 cup raw = one serving size)

Avocado = the best fast food on Earth	Rich in vitamins A, B complex, C, E, K and folate. Minerals: magnesium, copper, iron, calcium, potassium. More protein than cow's milk, all 18 amino acids, 7 fatty acids inc omega 3 & 6. Plenty of fiber. When you eat quality fat your cravings vanish.	Water content 65-80%, nutritional powerhouse. Slice in half, shake a little sea salt, or a bit of olive oil and balsamic vinegar or lemon, eat. Add to salads, sandwiches!
Beans	High in protein, complex carbohydrates. Contain both soluble and insoluble fiber, phytochemicals, protease inhibitors that may help prevent cancer.	(see Protein section, Chapter 1)
Beets	Their folic acid (a B vitamin) is crucial to DNA synthesis so healthy cells stay healthy, lowers risk of atherosclerosis, works against heart disease.	Boil or bake in foil till fork can puncture skin. Blend as color-ful juice. Add quinoa & spinach for uber-nutritional salad.
Broccoli	Contains more vitamin C (promotes wound healing, improves blood sugar levels for diabetes) than citrus, A, beta carotene, B-vitamins, chlorophyll, fiber, powerful antioxidants (see cruciferous vegetables, below). Powerful agent against asthma. Deters cancer cell development.	Eat raw, or steam until brightly colored, stir fry slightly. Squirt with Braggs amino acids for added protein and flavor! Squeeze lemon, mmm, fresh!

Cabbage, green or red	Heals peptic ulcer, excellent for detoxification of blood, constipation.High in phyto-nutrients, which lower risk of cancer in the lungs, prostate, colon, breasts, ovaries and bladder. Red cabbage: safeguard against Alzheimer's disease, has more phytonutrients than green. Excellent source of Vitamin C, calcium, fiber, manganese.	Eat raw, or drink the juice. Mix into stir frys. Add to salads and sandwiches, brown rice or quinoa.
Carrots: 2 carrots every other day provide enough beta carotene to reduce the risk of stroke by half for men who already have symptoms of heart disease[3]	Reduce the risk of cancer, strong eyes, healthy skin, prevent macular degenera-tion, heart disease. High in antioxidants; alkaline pH protects against acne and aging. Body converts carrot's beta-carotene into vitamin A: allows us to see in dim light. Boosts immunity, keeps respiratory system working optimally.	Raw: eat the "belly button" = most nutritious part! Stir into stovetop mixed veggies. Shred into salad, with light olive oil/balsamic vinegar, drink as juice
Chilli Peppers	Capsaicin, the heat source in chilis is an antioxidant. Contains blood thinning properties to prevent strokes, lowers cholesterol, protects DNA against carcinogens.	Add to stir fry, corn bread, wherever you want to kick up flavor
Cruciferous vegetables: cabbage, broccoli, kale, cauliflower, bok choy	High in phytonutrients, work to disarm free radicals before they damage DNA, cells, fat molecules such as cholesterol.	Eat raw, or steam until color is bright.
Garlic	Healing herb with antibiotic properties. Inhibits common cold virus. May lower blood pressures and cholesterol; protects from heart disease. Contains more than 30 different anti-carcinogens; may deter liver damage. Wards off mosquitos; athlete's foot remedy; fights funguses and parasites.	Sautée with olive oil whenever lightly cooking vegetables. Add to quinoa, brown rice, eggs, soups, salads, sauces – anywhere, is hugely beneficial!

Green and red peppers	High in vitamin C, a natural antihistamine (if you're stuffed up, eat peppers!). Promote wound healing, t-cell production, lower risk of cataracts.	Sautée with garlic, onions, tomatoes. Eat raw alone or in salads. Blend into soup.
Mushrooms	Contain beta-glucan, which stimulates immune system. Shitake, enoki, zhuling and reishi all have anti-cancer and antiviral effects. Anti-biotic properties increase white blood cell count, decrease fat and blood cholesterol. Promote longevity. Great source of potassium, riboflavin, niacin and selenium.	Sautée in olive oil or unsalted butter. Eat raw, add to salads. Blend into soup. Add to quinoa, brown rice, eggs, rice pasta, stir frys.
Onions	Allylic sulfides contain more than 30 different anti-carcinogens linked to liver, stomach, and lung cancers. Antioxidants inhibit growth of bacteria and viruses.	Sautée with peppers and zucchini; eat with brown rice or quinoa. Add to eggs.
Root vegetables, winter squashes	Influence the spleen, pancreas and stomach, improve energy and circulation. Excellent source of natural sugars, beta-carotene, carbohydrates. Perfect choice for diabetics and those with digestive problems. Beets, carrots and burdock are liver-cleansing foods.	Coat slightly with olive oil; roast in oven till tender. Chop and boil, puree into soup.
Soybeans and tofu**	Lower "bad" LDL cholesterol in bloodstream reducing the risk of heart disease.	(see Protein section) Mix into stir fry; add grilled cubes to salad, use as scrambled eggs.
Tomatoes	Contain vitamins A & C and lycopene, a potent anti-oxidant. Detoxifier: tonifies the stomach and cleans the liver. Stimulates immune function, may slow degen-erative diseases. Believed to contain up to 10,000 phytochemicals, active agents against cancer and disease.	Eat raw as salad, add to sandwiches, eggs. Sautée in olive oil with onion, peppers, zucchini, eggplant. Blend into soup. Add to quinoa, brown rice.

ORGANIC VEGGIES? WORTH A FEW MORE DOLLARS

A comparison of the nutritional content of organic and conventional, factory farmed vegetables indicates that organic produce contains higher nutritional value. Organic lettuce showed 29% more magnesium; organic spinach had 52% more vitamin C; organic carrots had 69% more magnesium and organic cabbage had 43% more vitamin C, 41% more iron and 40% more magnesium.[4]

**A few words about SOY. We used to eat soy and drink soymilk, and one day noticed the sugar content in soymilk. Then started paying attention to the many vegans and vegetarians whose diets were largely comprised of soy foods: soy burgers, soy bacon, soy cheese... After investigating we stopped eating unfermented soy altogether. Soy side effects include gas, bloating, "moobs" (man boobs), a host of thyroid problems, endocrine disorders, a range of menstrual abnormalities, puberty before age ten, hair loss and more. The trouble with soy is, as a result of farming subsidies it is present in everything from meat to chocolate to oil. Most soy (+94%) in this country is genetically modified.

Soy is a major allergen; it contains goitrogens which damage the thyroid; lectins, which cause red blood cells to lump together and may trigger abnormal immunity responses; oxalates, which prevent calcium absorption, cause painful kidney stones and vulvodynia, a vaginal disorder; isoflavones, lauded as natural estrogens, are serious endocrine disruptors, lowering testosterone, causing menstrual disorders, and cancer cell proliferation.[5]

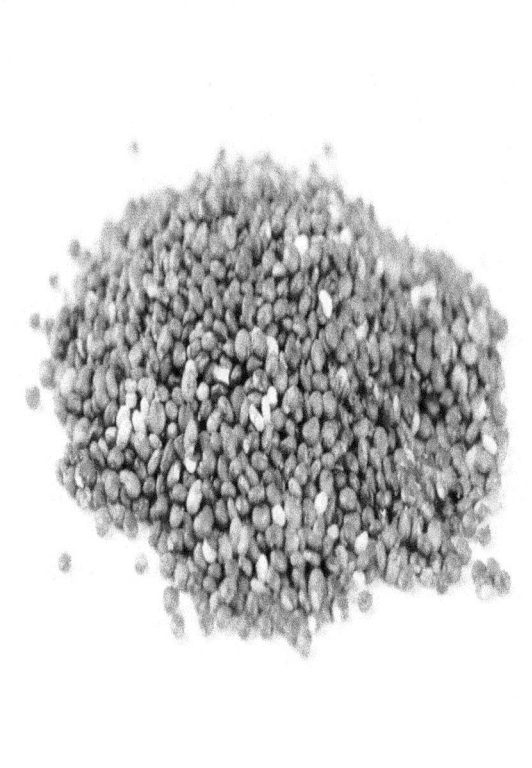

Gratifying Grains

I remember as child growing up in Detroit my mother filling the kitchen with bread after returning from the grocery store. She bought the usual sandwich bread: white and white painted brown with molasses. She also brought home a lot of bakery breads: buns and sweet rolls, sourdough, Hawaiian, bagels – always tons, so many, and so many of us in the family unconcerned with the root of the desire. We focused more on the need; when hungry, you could easily pull it apart and shove into your mouth without anyone questioning you. There wasn't a time of day that you couldn't eat bread; it had a connection to every meal and even in between. The sweet ones you could eat alone. The plain ones you just needed to add jam, butter or another condiment. Now, all this bread stands out to me now. The many arrays covering the kitchen counter seemed to suggest a theory my mother, as if she were an aspiring baker's apprentice or bread scientist of some sort. But now I realize after years of observing my family's eating habits, that this was probably an attempt at attacking the negative daily effects of simple carbohydrates.

All of that bread we consumed was devoid of important nutritional value. But how would we ever know or care when we had the busyness of our day in front of us, or we were distracted first by the traveling sugary highs and lows. There were plenty of companies pushing their incessant marketing and a willingness to support this eat-eat-eat behavior.

My brother and I were respectively heading to 6ft and my mother was trying to fill our growing structures. What we as a family did not know—did not know was how to interpret to our bodies cry for nutrients. What is their purpose? And just how many are there? For example, there's millet, kasha, brown rice and quinoa just to name a few. We could never have loaded ourselves three times a day with stone ground whole wheat and then had a little quinoa for dinner. Whole grains are much higher in fiber than white breads. They also include vitamin B6 and E, magnesium, zinc, folic acid and chromium. The quinoa alone has 50% more protein than wheat. You may not understand what these ingredients do when they enter the body. For now, eating grains can be understood in one simple way: 'less money at the grocery store'. If my mother had been feeding her two growing boys high-nutrient ingredients which take more time to break-down in the body – this would indeed have slowed the assault on the kitchen.

Adjusting to nutritious foods will take time; you will need to incorporate these foods slowly. You might have mouths that are used to sweetened grains, not looking for food to be so intelligent. **But in the end you will see that food that can save your life.**

It must begin with you. Once you properly understand the importance of this, you will better equipped to pass it on to your loved ones. When what you eat makes you feel good, you'll want those you love to feel good too.

When in the grocery store, spend a little more time looking for your grains. This can easily be overwhelming when it comes to bread, with its huge variety and ingredient lists. Companies realize that a confusing label can result in buying their products out of rush and frustration. Slow down and read the labels!

Unless you are gluten intolerant, always look for bread that states **whole wheat flour as the 1st ingredient**. Those that list wheat flour or *enriched* wheat flour are refined. This means the nutritious natural elements have been removed and chemically replaced.

Once you change shopping habits, reading labels will be the first empowering stage towards health and wellness. You will soon impulsively know which products to avoid and which to grab.

Grains were commonly eaten as whole grains until the last century. Advances in the milling and processing of grains allowed separation and removal of the bran and germ. This way it was more appealing to people's taste buds with its overall softer texture and extended freshness (shelf life). Yet, this is where the problem began. In the refining process most of the bran and some of the germ is removed, resulting in the loss of fiber, B vitamins, vitamin E, trace minerals, unsaturated fat and about 75 percent of the phytochemicals that boost the immune system with anti-inflammatory, antiviral, antibacterial and cellular repair. *"Enriched flour" means the vitamins are artificially processed back into the flour after stripping the grains' inherent vital nutrients.* A whole grain is made up of three key parts: the bran, the germ, and the endosperm. You will see it listed as whole, cracked, split, flaked or ground. Regardless of how the whole grain is sliced and diced, whole grain food delivers approximately the same proportions of bran, germ, and endosperm found in the original grain.

Names of Whole Grains

Whole Wheat, Millet Whole Oats, Popcorn, Whole Grain, Cornmeal, Quinoa, Brown Rice, Sorghum, Whole Rye, Amaranth, Whole-Grain, Barley, Emmer, Wild Rice, Farro, Buckwheat, Grano, Triticale, Spelt, Bulgar (Cracked Wheat), Groats

---

Whole grains contain: valuable anti-oxidants, essential enzymes, B vitamins, vitamin E, magnesium, iron, fiber, protein

What does this mean?

By eating 3 servings a day, with the phytochemicals and antioxidants in whole grains, can reduce your risk of:

- heart disease (by 25-36%)

- stroke (by 37%)

- cancer (digestive system by 21-43%, hormone related by 10-40%)

- diabetes (Type II by 21-27%)

- obesity[6]

Fiber plays a key role in healthy eating. Dietary fiber refers to the indigestible part of a carbohydrate food. Fiber is found in whole grain cereals, fruit (fresh and dried) and vegetables. A good intake of dietary fiber can prevent many digestive problems and protect against diseases like colon cancer and diverticular disease, as it improves the functioning of the intestines and encourages helpful bacterial growth in the colon. High-fiber foods accelerate food metabolism (burn calories 40% faster) and assist with weight loss. Fiber also helps to lower blood cholesterol (reducing the risk of heart disease) and stabilize blood sugar levels. A guideline for daily minimum fiber intake is 25 grams.

Gluten Intolerance

When talking grains there is no a way to continue without discussing gluten. Gluten is the protein component of wheat, rye and barley and for those allergic to wheat, or having digestive discomfort without knowing why, this could eventually cause Celiac disease, a chronic digestive disorder. This disease is inherited and affects 1 out of 133 Americans (most commonly Caucasians of European ancestry – women more than men). People today have so many digestive issues and often chalk them up to an overall general side effect of eating. But it is important for us to be accountable for our health, learn to get our ear closer to what our bodies are trying to say and begin to be honest with ourselves. There is a lot of opportunity for knowledge without taking medication or involving a professional.

If a person is gluten-intolerant and consumes gluten this gradually damages the small intestines. When gluten enters the body it causes the lining of the intestines to swell, and the intestines' tiny hair-like projections called villi begin to flatten with damage. This impairs the body's ability to absorb vital nutrients. The loss of vitamins, minerals and calories results in malnutrition. Just think about that for a moment. For example, vitamin A promotes healthy surface linings of respiratory, urinary and intestinal tract. Vitamin B6 helps to maintain your blood glucose. These vitamins play a vital role in your health – just imagine if they, along with many others, can't perform. The body begins to slowly deteriorate, for some. For others—based on their constitution—the body may deteriorate quickly. Here you have an opportunity to begin to feel better by simply removing this ingredient from your diet.

Common symptoms include abdominal swelling (feeling bloated after eating) constipation, cramps, loss of appetite and menstrual irregularities, nausea, fatigue, irritability, and depression. No, these are not the side effects of a popularly marketed drug. This is your body saying it has a problem with what you just ate. Many of these symptoms may be linked to other disorders. You could easily get yourself distracted by speculation from other family and friends, commercials, and bus stop ads, but you must begin to separate them.

Let's take for instance that last symptom: *abdominal swelling*. My friend had this problem for as long as she could remember. Doctors diagnosed this as irritable bowl syndrome, which was exactly one of the things going on: her bowels were irritated, her intestines were irritated. But what was really going on? When was this occurring? Were specific products causing this? What could she do to naturally alleviate her problem? These are questions she could have further pursued, but a diagnosis, a pamphlet and the comfort relayed by a professional, may send you on your way. Sometimes we don't want to get to the root of the problem, until the problems become exacerbated, and even then we just give it up to a professional, completely over-whelmed.

You may be someone with cancer, diabetes, or high blood pressure, loaded with so much information you don't know where to turn. You may want to test yourself for gluten intoler-ance and you may realize that removing one branch removes many other trees of separate, but related, problems. This action puts the power in your hands and may foster more comfortable evenings around food, family and friends.

Try this test:

Eliminate all gluten for one week: no bread, no pasta, no pizza, no cereal, nothing containing gluten.

On day 8 reintroduce it at your previous usage.

If, after eating you feel foggy, bloated, fatigued: you likely have an intolerance to gluten.

Gluten-Free Shopping

Sounds like a lot, right? Take your time. Start by incorporating **gluten free** products into your kitchen. Discover or rediscover what they taste like, and then move to substituting them for your commonly purchased items.

Key words to watch out for: wheat, barley, rye and oats, and: farina, flour, caramel coloring, enriched flour, cereal, hydrolyzed vegetable protein, malt flavoring or extracts, matzo, MSG, modified food starch, emulsifiers, stabilizers, distilled vinegar, seitan, semolina, spelt, durum, and triticale. All of these contain gluten.

Excellent Gluten-Free Grain Substitutes

Amaranth This ancient Aztec grain is rich in high-quality protein and lysine, plus dietary fiber, dietary minerals, iron, magnesium, copper, phosphorus, and especially manganese.

Buckwheat (Kasha) Hearty and filling! Has high concen-trations of most essential amino acids: lysine, theorinine, tryptophan; it also contains zinc, iron and selenium.

Quinoa (pronounced 'keenwa') Delicious, fast cooking grain, high in protein (50% more than wheat), iron, magnesium, phosphorous. Has the highest nutritional profile of all grains, consumed for thousands of years in South America.

Millet Nearly 15% protein high amounts of fiber, B-complex vitamins including niacin, thiamin, riboflavin, and essential amino acids. Millet is high in minerals: iron, magnesium, phosphorous, and potassium. Soothing: great for nausea or morning sickness; anti-fungal: Candida comfort.

These are definitely superfoods! They can be eaten for breakfast, lunch and dinner in many variations. From pancakes with buck-wheat to oatmeal. Or, in place of rice, quinoa. These products are in your grocery store. Take the time to learn more about them; they can be an important addition to your diet.

Others include products that specify gluten free. Here are some useful websites for further information.

www.glutenfree.com
www.bobsredmill.com/glutenfree
(also look for this company's line of products. Key wheat flour re-placements are rice, corn meal, tapioca, and potato.)

www.livingwithout.com
www.specialtyfoodshop.com

Dairy
& Moo-Juice Alternatives

In America, many of us grew up awash in milk and milk products before we could determine if this was best for our bodies.
For my family it was considered a prime source of vitamin D.
Milk was at the table for every meal. Milk was poured in our
cereal in the morning, at lunch I drank a glass or carton. Milk
was consumed again for dinner in meals like macaroni and
cheese, chicken casserole or mushroom soup. Even when you
eat a bag of chips or crackers, milk may be a by-product or
listed as a milk culture.

Are milk and milk products bad for you? You can't come to
these decisions through TV commercials or a marketing cam-
paign, rather, you have to listen to what your body says. After
leaving my parents' home, I started to eat differently and eventually realized whole milk and certain yellow cheeses weren't right
for me. Was I lactose intolerant (lacking the enzyme lactase that
allows for proper digestion of dairy products)? I wasn't completely sure, but eventually I found goat or sheep cheeses
digested more easily for me. Is it because these animals are
mostly grass eaters? Possibly. Does this mean I can eat products
from cows that are grass fed? Another possibility.

This sort of investigation leads to better health and less distraction with food. No one else can tell you how your body feels.

This you must determine on your own, and by doing so you will not sacrifice your bodies' desires or the nutrients you need. You ultimately will adjust your selection process to one that is more of a balance and unique to your own body and its history.

Humans are the only mammals to continue to drink milk after infancy, and the milk of another species. Many cultures, such as in Asia and Africa, historically never drank milk and often have difficulty digesting it. Some ethnic groups do not have the enzymes to digest milk. Despite the omnipresent campaigns to drink it, cow's milk is the #1 allergic food in the U.S.

LACTOSE INTOLERANT: 50 million Americans

- 90% Asian Americans

- 74% Latino Descent

- 80% African Americans

- 15% Caucasian

Are you lactose intolerant? While not causing as debilitating problems as with Celiac disease, this does create gastrointestinal problems such as stomach cramps, gas, nausea, bloating and diarrhea as well as acne.

As with gluten, test your tolerance this way: eliminate all dairy for one week. Reintroduce on day 8 at normal consumption. See above symptoms to determine your tolerance after 30 minutes - 2 hours.

Does drinking milk actually *cause* bone loss? Does it lead to cancer, heart disease, obesity, diabetes, breast and prostate cancer? Perhaps you have heard how "factory farm" animals are being inhumanely treated? Would all of this prompt you to stop drinking milk? In many cases the answer would be no because these ideas are repeatedly being stated yet millions continue to consume it and surround their decisions with their own logic. I am not here to tell you if you should or shouldn't drink milk, but rather to ask you to look at your ancestry and also realize that there are unnatural additives in factory-farmed diary products. If your family member has a chronic disease you have to be more diligent. Above all, listen to your body.

If you are removing cow's milk from your diet and find this daunting, try some of these alternatives: rice, almond or hemp milk. Try these in food such as cereal or in baking where the taste can be offset. Choose real butter, you can't go wrong (in moderation, of course).

Remember, there are milk cultures in many snack foods as well: **read the ingredients.**

Most important: notice how you feel.

What to look for instead: Organic or raw milk*/cheese, butter, goat and sheep milk/cheeses, rice milk, hemp milk, almond milk/cheese, oat milk, ghee, yogurt

---

Check your local farmers market for freshly prepared milk, cream, butter, cheese and yogurt. See if you can find raw milk products in your region[8]. Seek out unhomogenized milk. During homogenization, at high pressure, milk is sent through a tiny filter, breaking up the fat so it is evenly dispersed in the milk. The end result, while lasting longer, has questionable health repercussions.[9]

Dairy is highly mucus producing. If you're on a cleansing diet or feeling stuffed up, or if your nose is always running, it may be due to your consumption of dairy products. Dairy foods can burden the respiratory, digestive and immune systems.

* Raw milk is a controversial topic. Pasteurization sterilizes the milk and enhances shelf life, yet, this heating process also destroys all bacteria and enzymatic activity. Cows in this country are fed diets heavy in grain (corn), soybeans and cottonseed meal–this milk requires pasteurization to protect from pathogenic infection. Fresh, organic grass-fed milk has natural bactericidal ingredients and antibiotic properties to stifle unwanted microbial growth. Raw milk from grass-fed cows is a complete and balanced food. Some say you could live on it and nothing else for the rest of your life. Fresh raw milk will last from 7-10 days refrigerated. All raw milk is not created equal! Know the source, aim for predominantly grass-fed, preferably organic, animals.

Almond milk	Made by soaking & pressing ground almonds with pure water. Cholesterol-free, more protein and iron, and less calories than cow's milk.	Use wherever you would use milk; go for unsweetened versions.
Ghee	Clarified butter; here, milk proteins are separated and removed, leaving only the fat of the butter. Ghee is very stable and does not need refrigeration, will last in your pantry for over a year. Used in Indian culture for centuries.	Prized for its buttery flavor, it can be used in stir-fries, on steamed veggies, melted on freshly popped popcorn, or in baking.
Yogurt	Intestinal cleanser, balances and replaces friendly flora in the G.I. tract. Nutrient-dense with proteins, more calcium than milk, vitamins, minerals. Lowers bad cholesterol, strengthens against osteoporosis, will decrease diarrhea in children.	Aim for unprocessed, unsweetened, plain yogurt such as Greek yogurt or Fage brand, not flavored or "low fat". Add fruit and chopped raw almonds, or granola.
Kefir	Complete protein. Contains biotin, B vitamins (+B12), calcium, magnesium. Used in treating metabolic and gastric disorders, allergies, atherosclerosis. Replenishes beneficial intestinal bacteria, balances stomach pH.	Simply drink up. Not lactose-free.

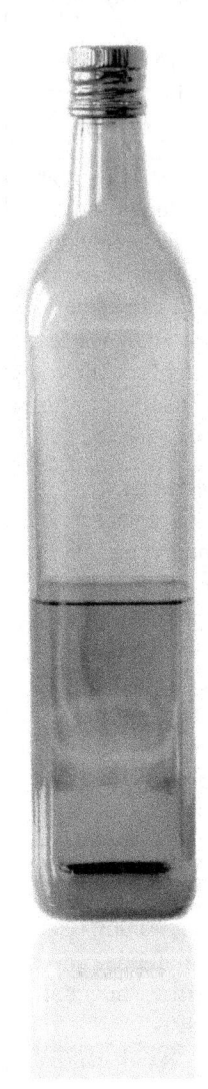

Fats & Oils

Nothing to Fear

We know what bad fats are. Our weight gain and poor digestion tell us. In the last half of the 20th century, Americans increased their fat intake by over 33%! Many successful companies have done an excellent job volunteering for this co-conspiracy. In store aisles, for example, they are almost screaming at us through their colorful packaging and health claims. I could easily single out products that have caused problems for me and I'm sure you can as well, but to really own the experience of what is a good and bad fat, we will have to discover this by eating good fats and comparing. Only then can our bodies properly argue the case for our minds. I find that this is how a true consensus can be achieved, over small and big advertising dollars. Your own self-discovery fuels it.

The healthy fats are monounsaturated, found in nuts, such as peanuts, walnuts, almonds and pistachios; also included are avocado and olive oil. Polyunsaturated fats are also healthy, including seafood like salmon and fish oil as well as corn, soy, safflower and sesame and flax oils. Omega3 is also included here. Saturated fat is technically the bad fat—most of its fat comes from animal products such as meat, dairy, eggs and seafood such as lobster. The oils in this group include coconut, palm and palm kernel.

Finally the trans fats, the worst form of fat, has been scientifically created through hydrogenating liquid oils. These fats give more shelf life to many of our favorite snack foods, are in vegetable shortening, margarine and a lot of fast food chains. Trans fats have been linked to cancer risk, lowered immune response, impaired cell function and premature skin aging. They interfere with the metabolism of natural fats. Attempt to avoid these and begin to discover new loves with real snacks.

Choosing oils will take a little time at first. The extensive variety of oils on store shelves can be daunting. From the list that we provide, take a little time selecting the ones you will be using. When it comes to olive oil, know that there are different grades. You will see virgin, extra virgin, first cold press etc. Remember to find one that works for your body and budget (they can be priced anywhere from 5 to 60 dollars) and keep experimenting through trial and error. Do what I do: go for the one that tastes best to you. As a stand alone, olive oil has a very important nutritional value. You will find yourself getting more familiar with it and its positive impact on your foods and in your body.

One last note: trans fat has given saturated fat a bad name. Since its inception it has proceeded to attack the health of many of us through increased health complications. Some saturated fats such as red meat, cheese, butter and real yogurt could properly support a fat daily allowance via nutrients and good intestinal bacteria. In some cases, this type of fat has to be completely avoided because of what it has done to our bodies. It will take time to first heal the inflammation through eating proper foods before you can return to a better balance of fats. Again, take on the responsibility of listening to your body.

THE GOOD FATS

MONOUNSATURATED	*For anyone suffering from a chronic disease, first pressed olive oils for cooking are recommended.*
Olives Olive oil (extra virgin or first press) Grape Seed oil (organic) Avocados	Fat from high-quality oils and whole foods helps keep metabolism steady, nourish our skin, hair and nails, and keep healthy "grease in our engine" for fluid body functions.
Almonds (raw) (on a weight loss program, eat nuts sparingly)	Of all the nuts, highest in calcium and fiber, great source of high-quality fatty acids, protein.
Cashews (raw)	High in protein, minerals: iron, magnesium, phosphorus, zinc, copper and manganese
Pecans (raw) (60% monounsaturated)	High in iron, contain 19 vitamins and minerals, 18% protein, high in phytochemicals
POLYUNSATURATED	
Safflower oil Cottonseed oil Fish, for omega 3s, especially salmon, canned sardines (bones intact), tuna	Contain omega-3 fatty acids: reduce effects of harmful fat & cholesterol. Omega-3s: essential to human health, reduce risk of blood clots, abnormal heart rhythms, arterial plaque and lower blood pressure. 7-10 oz of fish (salmon, mackerel, sardine) per week is sufficient.
Walnuts (raw)	Use to strengthen kidney, lungs: brain food. Nuts & seeds help build the body, have grounding effect; rich in nutrients, minerals, such as vitamin E, selenium*.
Flaxseed	53% omega-3 fatty acid
Pumpkin seeds	Extremely high in protein and EFAs; rich in zinc, iron and calcium. 15% omega 3s. Cook with grains and vegetables, toast with light sea salt.

*Selenium, an antioxidant mineral responsible for tissue elasticity, protects the skin from damage from excessive ultraviolet light and also prevents cell damage by free radicals. Selenium is correlated with a reduction of breast cancer risk. Dietary sources of selenium include wheat germ, seafood such as tuna and salmon, garlic, Brazil nuts, eggs, brown rice, and whole-wheat bread. Brazil nuts are perhaps the best source: 3-4 per day provides adequate selenium for most people.

THE NOT GOOD FATS

SATURATED (use sparingly)	
Whole milk Ghee Butter Cheese Ice cream Animal protein Chocolate Coconut oil, milk	For those not suffering from inflammation, some saturated fat is not bad. Butter is better for you than margarine; animal protein also, if it's from free-roaming, grass-fed, antibiotic-free animals. Coconut oil is a good cooking oil and source of lauric acid, disease-fighting fatty acid.
TRANS FAT (avoid)	Trans fat should be completely avoided by all.
Fried fast foods Most commercially produced food (read labels)	Heavily processed. Our bodies do not metabolize these well.
Baked goods unless homemade (check ingredients)	"partially hydrogenated oil" means trans fat

The skinny on FATS.

Our bodies need fat. Fat is our most reliable source of fuel, providing twice the energy of carbohydrates or protein. Fat lubricates the skin and hair, and protects body tissues and organs and against the cold. Fat makes hormones and is necessary for the assimilation of the fat-soluble vitamins A, D, E and K. Fats supply essential fatty acids and deliver vital nutrients to the nervous system.

Cholesterol is an essential fat made by the liver and necessary for good health. Essential for the production of cell membranes and hormones, our bodies produce all the cholesterol it needs. Additional cholesterol comes from eating meat and dairy, and fatty foods. Excess amounts will accumulate on arterial walls and reduce the body's ability to manage blood pressure changes. Stiff and narrow arteries create greater demands on the heart, putting it at risk over time.

Essential fatty acids (EFAs) are healthy fats that protect our bodies from degenerative and cardiovascular disease and boost our brainpower. They maintain energy, insulate our bodies, are responsible for skin repair, moisture content, and overall flexibility, but because the body cannot produce its own EFAs, they must be obtained through the diet. EFAs reduce the risk of breast and colon cancer, and reduce inflammation of rheumatoid arthritis and osteoarthritis. Dry, inflamed skin or skin that suffers from the frequent appearance of whiteheads or blackheads can benefit from supplementing omega-3 fatty acids. Children with attention deficit disorder have been found to lack EFAs.

Beware of foods labeled "low-fat" as they are higher in sugar (which if not used, gets stored as fat and trigger the insulin roller coaster).

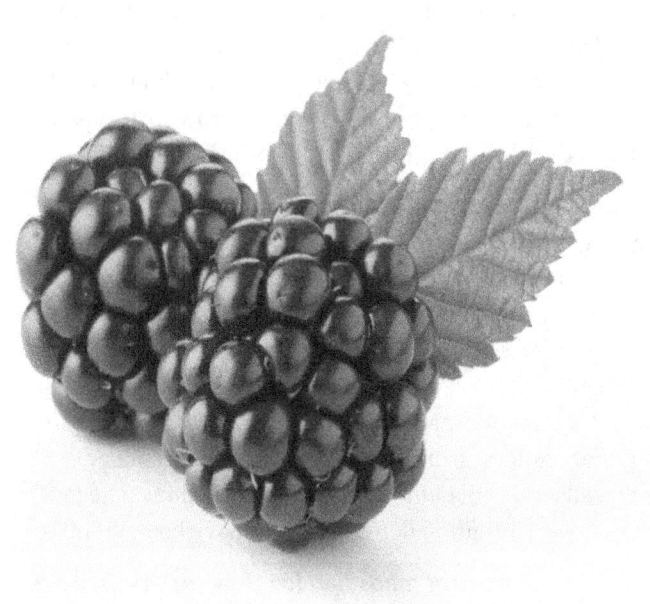

Fruits

Fruits, especially berries, make everything better

For many of us eating a variety of fruits it is not something we have to be forced to do. Of course fruit is also presented to us in variations, such as with sugar, in pies, in syrup, in juices and with whipped cream. The core nutrients are lost as the fruit is turned into a dessert. My relationship with fruit has changed in the last few years. Fruit, for me, has become a bit of a stand alone—far more than a dessert, or a bridge in between meals. I have discovered fruit in a nutritious and medicinal way.

I eat apples, grapefruits, pears, cherries, peaches, etc. because I desire them—my body desires the healing powers of these fruits. It needs them to do everything from aiding intestinal swelling to treating anemia. Fruit is working for us, it's on the job. Just behind its skin—its soft, sweet and sometimes sour juiciness— it reveals its gentle ploy.

Apples with their fiber, grapefruit with their fever reduction, grapes with their benefits to the kidneys; these add up to much more than an afternoon snack. If you listen closely—real closely-you will hear your body asking you for a specific fruit: watermelon in the summertime because of its cooling, thermal nature, oranges for their treatment of colds in the winter. As you enjoy it with a friend, fruit will treat your thirst, remedy your constipation, lower your high blood pressure and treat your urinary difficulties. Fruit can be extremely effective.

While some fruits might keep things flowing, berries work more in prevention. Berries are superfoods* that continue to play second fiddle. For example, cranberries can protect you from periodontal gum disease, cancer and heart disease. Blueberries are high in antioxidants that fight against free radicals. Strawberries reduce the risk of certain cancers. To include more berries in your diet, consider blending them into a shake in the morning or a spilling handful over your cereal.

Remember that fruit is more than snack; it is a healing superfood.

*Generally, fruits and vegetables given a 'superfood' tag are high in antioxidants such as vitamin C, flavonoids (found in citrus fruits and berries), and other phytochemicals (biologically active non-nutrient components that give them color, flavor an natural disease resistance) such as beta-carotene, are also known for their antioxidant properties, which is why brightly colored fruit and vegetables are considered especially beneficial. Because antioxidants are especially effective at combating free radicals (harmful molecules that damage cells and DNA and can contribute to aging, heart disease and cancer) they make fruit and vegetables particularly good for health.

WHY EAT FRUITS? As nutrient-dense healers, the more fruits you eat, the less your risk of disease. Their flavonoids keep cancer-causing hormones from attaching to cells. Fresh fruits accelerate cleansing and help alkalize the body. Their natural water and natural sugar provide quick energy and speed up the calorie-burning process. Best eaten fresh; when cooked their properties become acid-forming. Some absorb pesticides more (peaches, pears, nectarines, apples: choose organic). Others, because skins are removed before eating (bananas), are less impacted. One serving is 1 medium piece of fruit or 6 oz of fresh squeezed juice (not pasteurized).

THE BERRIES

What	Why	How
Blackberries	These have the highest antioxidant capacity of all fruits.10 Excellent source of vitamins A, B, C, E, calcium, iron, especially fiber.There is as much vitamin C in six flavonoid-packed blackberries as in one lemon.	Fresh, if possible; if frozen, go organic. In smoothies, yogurt, as breakfast, snack or dessert.
Blueberries	The food with the highest antioxidant activity; may be helpful in improving memory function and healthy aging. Top source of flavonoids.	Fresh, if possible. If frozen, organic. In smoothies, yogurt, as breakfast or dessert
Cranberries	High in antioxidants and phytonutrients; helpful in preventing urinary tract infections, also helpful in protecting from heart disease, cancer, stomach ulcers, periodontal gum disease.	Be sure to read the label on juice and beware of additives.
Strawberries	Source of essential vitamins and minerals: vitamin C, folate, fiber, potassium and antioxidants. Contain ellagic acid, holds anti-cancer properties.	Eat organic, if possible, as these are hard hit with many varieties of pesticides.

OTHER FRUITS[11]

Apples	Contain ellagic acid, an anti-carciogen for skin tumors and chemically induced cancers. High in fiber, especially apple skin.	Eat organic, if possible – apples are the hardest hit with a huge pesticide variety.
Apricots	Fresh apricots are high in beta-carotene, vitamin C and fiber, and alpha- carotene: inhibit tumor growth, powerful cancer preventer.	Choose organic when possible.
Bananas	Rich in magnesium: help protect circulatory system, potassium and slowly-absorbed sugars. Good source of pectin, a soluble fiber; aids digestion.	Try frozen with almond butter on sliced top. In cereal, smoothies, sautéed as dessert.
Cherries	Tart red cherries can relieve pain and inflammation. Excellent for remedying gout.	Eat 20 fresh daily, or frozen organic.
Citrus Fruits	Possess 58 known anti-cancer compounds, neu-tralize chemical carcinogens. Rich in bio-flavonoids, vitamin C: improve blood sugar levels in non-insulin dependent diabetics.	Enjoy fresh whenever possible. (concentrated and pasteurized juices lose much nutritional value in the process)
Currants	Source of anthocyanins, help relieve inflammation. Anti-oxidants promote healthy aging, neurological functions.	Add to yogurt, carrot salad, any baked goods.
Grapes	High in phytochemicals that aid in disease prevention and good health. Assist in healthy kidney functions.	Eat organic, if possible. Fresh or frozen.

Grapefruit	Vitamin C: antioxidant, antimicrobial, and Vitamin E: antioxidant. Fever reduction.	Whole fruit or fresh juice
Kiwis	Contain high amounts of enzymes, help combat autoimmune diseases, allergies, cancer and AIDS.	Whole fruit, great in smoothies, yogurt, salads
Mangos	Contain bioflavonoids that aid the immune system.	Slice into shake with almond milk, yum!
Oranges	Contain glutathione, a potent antioxidant confirmed to combat disease. Rich in beta-carotene and vitamin C. Most concentrated form of glucarate, a powerful cancer inhibitor.	Eat fresh only, directly from orange (com-mercially processed orange juice does not hold same properties)
Papayas	High amounts of enzymes help combat autoimmune diseases, allergies, as well as AIDS and cancer. Aids digestion.	Fresh or frozen, delicious in yogurt or smoothie.
Pineapples	Bromelain stimulates immune response; helps combat autoimmune diseases, allergies, cancer and AIDS. Bromelain also reduces inflammation, aids digestion.	Eat fresh only; delicious with fresh basil and pomegranate seeds.
Pomegranates	Deserve an entire chapter: benefit heart health, proven helpful in treating diabetes, dementia, cancer, meno-pausal issues. Anti-oxidant: reduces progression of high blood cholesterol. Relief from eczema, psoriasis, sunburn. Conjugated fatty acids: strong anti-inflammatory, reduce swelling, muscle aches and pains.	Seek out the pure juice, be sure to read label.

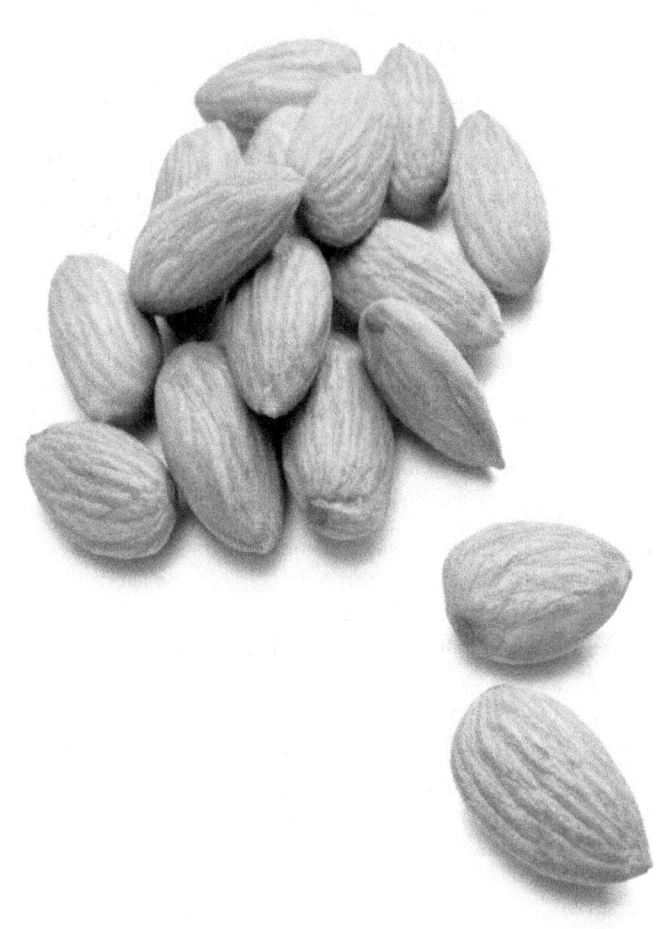

Snacks

The satisfying energy boost

I remember once being on the train heading out of town. It was a 5-hour ride and prior to departure we all sat in a waiting room and prepared ourselves. I watched a couple interchange bags of snacks. One of the bags was too small so they, with great care and a sense of enjoyment, put their snacks into a much larger one.

Once onboard, after we settled in I noticed this same couple sitting just across the aisle from me. Riding for an hour or so they slowly opened everything from snack crackers to pretzels dipped in chocolate. Sounds of excited conversation, laughter and more snacking emanated from their row and I found myself studying them. I started thinking about snacks and traveling. I knew if I had been with someone I would have been doing the same thing, and been much noisier. The only difference would have been the snacks chosen.

I know for sure that snacking goes with traveling and many other things in America. Snacks act as a catalyst and add to our enjoyment. There is something personally satisfying: traveling, watching TV, alone or communing with friends...all while eating your favorite snack. It promotes the purpose, whatever it is, the trip, the time together. Advertisers understand this completely. They need you and your kids to grow up with their brands. They need you to treat them as another one of your friends as they help sign off on your important moments. But let's look closer. Alarming rates of diabetes and heart disease, etc. are on the rise. The laughter doesn't stay for long – snacks are contributing to this epidemic.

What I personally have discovered, just like many others I'm sure, is that snacking has gone awry. Snacks have become dangerous with their lists of unpronounceable ingredients and their far too few nutrients. These foods have caused many problems with their chemicals and artificial flavorings. People who are struggling with their lives have started using them to prolong their despair rather than enhance their living. Entire communities in our country are suffering at the hands of poor quality snack foods being pushed in grocery stores. People living with better stores have deceptive advertisers confusing them because of their distracted busy lives.

Advertising has us thinking that it is all about the cartoon leopard on the bag, as if snack foods are the center of our travel or gatherings. As if the only reason you called up your friends and requested to see them was so you could ply yourselves with cheese puffs! The taste is so addicting that we have clouded our judgment with it. Food companies have seized this opportunity, just like any other American company with shareholders to please. Everything in this country is susceptible to becoming a no-holds-barred business.

Over the years your body may have slowly been taken over. For whatever reason, you may have eased into its new control. Maybe your diminishing health has set off alarms. But guess what? You are completely in charge of changing this. You can either do it through your own volition or with the help of a professional. Understand that there is no one to blame; most of the people who work at these companies find themselves subject to the same deceptive practices. Food, and particularly snack food, can be a great teacher: think while you reach for snacks. Ask yourself questions: am I awake or asleep? How do I want to feel: alive or deadened? Consider your relationships. Being in loving relationships means you are being love: not only to your mate and friends but also to your body. Take your next snacking opportunity to exemplify this. Try fresh figs, a handful of raw almonds, or hummus with carrots or rice crackers. Use this opportunity to put a stop to mindless eating. Free your mind from unhealthy dialogue, make choices that bring steady energy and peacefulness. This, you'll see, will also change the direction of your relationships.

As we begin exploring these issues we can help ourselves immensely if we read ingredient lists and look for suspects (listed below). This will reduce the body's turmoil and begin healing. You can heal, and allow wellness to spread to other parts of your life. Do not be afraid to ask for help (we will provide you with the best sources). I've watched my snacking over the years and noticed parallels with what was going on with my relation-ships. I've watched myself pouring through entire snack boxes looking for the missing nutrients that I didn't acquire in my meals. I also enjoyed the temporary comfort it gave me, or shelter from what was really going on in my life. While you are running a mental experiment on yourself with snacks, your body—as smart as it is—is looking for missing nutrients to help it function better. Once we get on the same game plan there is no question other parts of our life will improve.

Healthy Snacks

Often, once we're eating nutritious meals, we find our need for snacks becomes diminished or is eliminated altogether. This is another sign of approaching your ideal weight.

Drink a large glass of pure* water first. Usually, when we think we're hungry, we're actually thirsty.

Water is crucial to good health:

Drink ½ your body weight in ounces each day (we lose about a pint of water each day just breathing).

Water helps EVERYTHING.

THINK OF SNACKS AS *TEXTURAL* AND SATISFY *THAT* CRAVING. [12]

Sweet

- organic dark chocolate, 70% cacao: just a bit, delicious and satisfying!
- fresh, whole fruit, any kind
- sweet vegetables: carrots, sweet potatoes, yams, squashes – cut chunky, dash of olive oil and cinnamon, bake
- yogurt – full fat with fruit or honey
- apple or banana (frozen, yum!) with almond butter
- dried fruits – figs are filling and excellent source of fiber too!
- grass juice shot: wheatgrass or barley grass, mmm

- use leftover grains as porridge: add agave or maple syrup, nutmeg, cinnamon...add almond or rice milk and bananas, cranberries, etc.
- smoothies: mix what you have on hand: fruit, almond milk, yogurt, add ice, etc.
- "ice cream" fruit: peel a banana, freeze, blend in a food processor with nuts, berries, raisins or dates. Use frozen fruits like mango, papaya, berries!
- use juicer for carrot, apple, beet, celery, cucumber juices – add ginger!
- freshly squeezed citrus juices: make your own and try different combos
- sprouted date bread with natural jam or honey or almond butter

Creamy

- avocado: one a day keeps the doctor away
- yogurt: Greek or FAGE, go for full fat
- dips and spreads, like hummus, baba ganoush, guacamole
- soups: purees of vegetables. Cold soups are delicious too!
- mashed sweet potatoes, add parsnips and garlic, mmm!
- coconut milk and brown rice for rice pudding
- smoothies: add lots of fresh fruits

Crunchy

- nuts, always raw, not dry roasted. Almonds are best for energy, nutritive value

- plain organic popcorn, use olive oil to pop in a covered pan
- rice cakes, find with seaweed
- apples, organic: one a day, you'll feel great
- carrots, organic (not peeled)
- celery, organic, and dip (hummus, tabouli, favorite homemade dressing)
- celery and peanut butter or almond butter (use fresh pressed nut butters)
- grapes, fresh or frozen

Salty

- edamame with sea salt
- pickles and cornichons
- hummus, make your own, super easy and inexpensive
- oysters, sardines, pickled herring, smoked salmon
- steamed vegetables with tamari/shoyu
- make your own tortilla chips and guacamole or salsa, super easy!
- sauerkraut: eliminates sweet cravings
- olives, small handful of fresh ones (not canned)

*Pure water is h2O with all of the contaminants removed. Water from a household tap is generally municipal water. By law, **municipal water** supplies, upon request, will provide its customers a chemical analysis of their water composition. **Distilled water**, the most common form of pure water, is boiled and the steam is then condensed into a sanitary container in which the contaminants are left behind - does not guarantee a bacteria-free product unless the container is completely sterilized. (These waters are perfect for curling irons, clothes irons and steamers, humidifiers, and any appliance that requires water.) Bottled waters can include **artesian**: from a well that taps a confined aquifer (a water-bearing underground layer of rock or sand). **Mineral** waters contain not less than 250 parts per million total dissolved solids at the point of emergence from the source (these include iron, potassium, magnesium, manganese, silica, chromium, lithium, and copper). No minerals can be added. While these are healthful, the value of mineral waters versus spring waters is still debated. **Spring** water is derived from a natural underground formation where water flows to the surface. This water must be collected only at the spring.

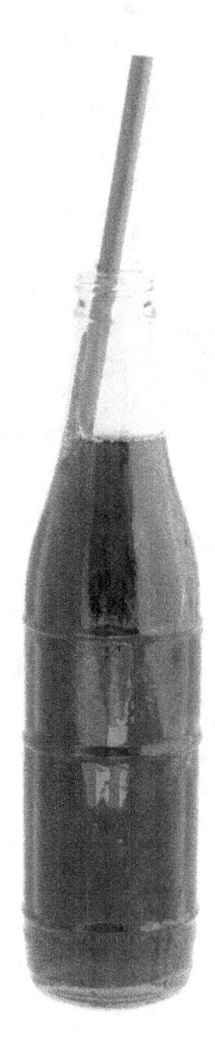

Inflammation

You're in Flames

Inflammation, the first sign of trouble in the body, is where most chronic diseases begin. Real killers such as heart disease, diabetes and cancer, as well as asthma and acid reflux. Symptoms take years in a poor habitat to create. Then various ailments appear, which you might dismiss as 'getting older' or it might provide you with a topic commiserate over with your friends.

Your doctor may have told you that: your weight gain, fluid in your legs, breathing problems, pain in your abdomen, joints, etc. is connected to one of the above diseases. You may settle down and relax into it, as if the case has been solved—but, in fact, this is only the beginning. Inflammation is an overall call to arms that requires your full attention.

The first thing we must understand about inflammation is that a lot of help is available. Start with a little reckoning in your own life. Get some knowledge about your own behavior.

When you review this book, a lot of you might notice your favorite foods are not mentioned. If they are, maybe accusations are being lobbed in their direction. This is because if inflammation exists, then there is surely stress, processed foods, sodas, 'fruit' drinks, candy bars, excessive animal fats and/or encased meats, fast foods, hard alcohol, coffee and smoking. If there is inflammation, your own behavior will have to be called into question: your relationship to these foods will have to be exposed.

Many of us are not accountable for our own experiences. Every symptom/problem that we have, we often try to quickly solve, based on someone else's experience. Seems like that would be logical, right? A friend of yours is suffering from a chronic disease that you are experiencing. You will of course ask him/her about the treatment to see if yours is similar. What you may find is that the doctor has prescribed the same drug. But are your nationalities, medical, family history, size and gender the same? Are you experiencing the same fears and/or anxieties?

Every human experience is unique regardless of how it looks, and the food we intake has different effects on us as well. Too many processed foods can change your health outcome to one that includes a chronic disease. So it will come down to what degree of its severity will you have, and when will it present itself? Some suffer in their teens, some as seniors. Some could lose their limbs; some could have a heart attack. Some develop colitis, diverticulitis and high blood pressure. You have some control over these outcomes.

Regardless of the "what" and the "when", the consistency of results is simple: it is all debilitating. Heredity can determine which ailment you are susceptible to, but you can influence the degree of its impact.

Growth hormones in milk or aspartame in soda could have different effects on someone whose parent has developed cancer. The additional sugar in low fat foods is going to have a different effect on someone whose family has a history of diabetes. But regardless, if the diabetes doesn't get you, or the heart disease, something debilitating will, if you continue eating poorly.

We cannot live free from ailments; we all will have them. The chronic ones, however, intensify discomfort in our lives. These need to be addressed. Natural foods or organic foods are going to save you from many of these problems. You are in charge, you must be accountable. But you are going to need some help. Processed food companies and advertisers are very clever and have embedded themselves deeply into our lives. They have created and marketed scientifically studied foods that are extremely tasty, addicting and dangerous. We can win though – not by dieting or avoidance, but changing our mindset. **Eating healthy is a habit just like eating poorly.** Creating that habit is where the help comes in, such as working with a holistic health counselor, nutritionist, or other trusted healing professional.

The addictions we have are complicated and unique from case to case. For many, working with someone may help to get to the root of the problem. When it comes to habit-forming, holistic health counselors, who address the unique situation of the whole person, know the way back from inflammation to wellness. We have been confronted with the complicated stories of clients who are eating a bag of chips for breakfast. Just like the one behind my daily king sized candy bar and soda, our stories need light. They may be culpable in the destruction of our health. If you do your part, your loving counselor will do his or hers. Together we will reinforce eating quality foods. Your counselor just needs your self-awareness and your willingness. In the meantime, plenty of fresh water, whole foods, regularly moving the body, and deep breathing go a long way in self-healing.

To prevent inflammatory conditions, eat a diet rich in wild fish, fresh fruits and vegetables, nuts, and seeds. Blueberries and cranberries provide polyphenolic protection against sight-damaging inflammation and oxidative stress. Cherries (the tarter the better!) are another inflammation-fighting food. Limit or eliminate red meat, alcohol, hydrogenated fats, refined sugars, and flours. Aim to avoid drinking soda. Whether diet or regular, soda brings acid reflux, kidney stones, softens your bones and creates an overly acidic digestive environment, leading directly to inflammation.

Evaluating and choosing the best natural anti-inflammatory depends on the specific condition, but the foremost herbal remedies include ginger, turmeric, boswellia, bromelain, glucosamine sulfate, omega-3 essential fats, slippery elm, fenugreek, and devil's claw root. Curcumin is the primary active anti-inflammatory component of turmeric. This plant contains antioxidant, anti-inflammatory, antiviral, and antifungal properties. Like ginger, it inhibits the enzymes and prostaglandins that play a role in inflammation.

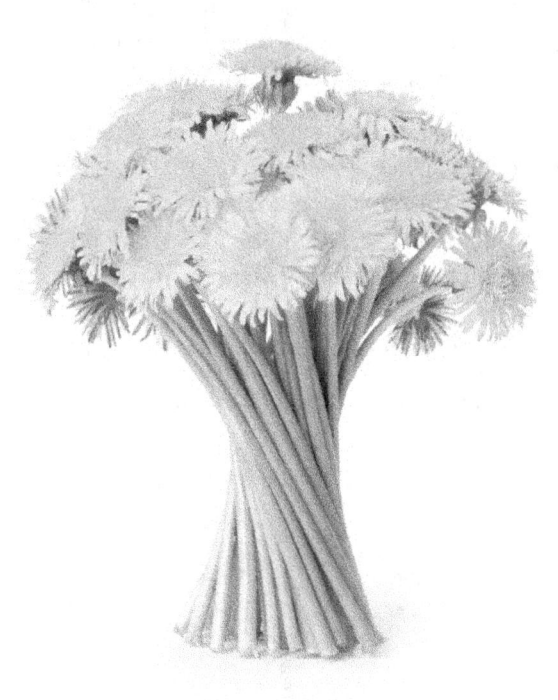

Epilogue

As Holistic Health Counselors, Joelle and I have worked across many clients in our various forms of practice who have, due to their health challenges or lack of nutritional understanding, inspired us to create this guide. As you may know, there are many books on healthy eating nowadays. Due to the soaring rates of obesity, heart disease and chronic illnesses in this country, we believe there can't be enough of these books.

What we've done here is not only present you with healthy choices but empower you as well. We provided the 'How, What and Why', but more importantly, helped you to understand how accountability factors into this process. **It's not just about making better choices, but also about finding your personal reasons for making better choices.** You shouldn't change to a healthy lifestyle because your family, doctor, mate wants you to. You want to, because you need to feel your best to be at your best.

As counselors we understand that you can't simply tell people to eat better. You can't just show them how to eat healthy. We have to help people to unearth their own reasons for being healthy. Willingness is key: then follows accountability.

What we have written here is a supermarket guide, a breakdown of food groups; we talk about why to eat certain foods, ways to prepare food and its inherent nutritional value. But what you will see inbetween the lines is our compassion for what really matters. And that is healing. Food heals, and consequently, what you are experiencing in your families, career, love relationships and exercise regimen gives way to a better life. That is the only thing that truly matters. That is the engine behind all of it. This book reminds you of something that you already know, something that you already feel deep down inside. **In the end you will find that you are in charge.**

Appendices

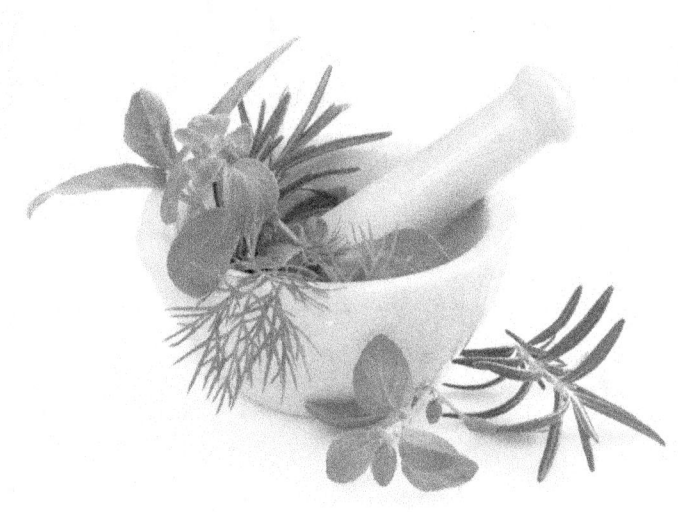

Prescriptive Remedies

Directory of Prescription Foods:
food solutions for common physical ailments.

R℞: Acne

Avoid diets high in saturated fats and animal products, including dairy. Avoid sugar and all processed foods. Eat a high-fiber diet, increase intake of raw foods containing oxalic acid such as almonds, beets, cashews and Swiss chard. Eat lots of fruits and foods rich in zinc: shellfish, soybeans, whole grains, sunflower seeds. Be sure your diet is rich in Vitamins A, C, E and essential fatty acids. Drink at least 8 glasses of quality water each day. Apple cider vinegar mixed with pure water (1:10 parts) can be applied to the affected area for relief and healing – or a paste of bentonite or other clay moistened with apple cider vinegar – leave on ½ hour and wash off with water.

R℞: Adrenal Fatigue

Your adrenal glands are situated just above your kidneys; under prolonged or extreme stress this area may become tender, or you may sweat excessively from little activity, have dark circles, muscle twitches or feel tired/wired. Avoid: alcohol, coffee, caffeine, soda (including diet!); dairy; dieting and long periods without food; fruit juices; preservatives, junk and processed food (inc. refined carbohydrates and white flour), fried foods, hydrogenated fats; skipping breakfast; sugar, sodium chloride. Include: Celtic sea salt or Himalayan salt to replenish electrolytes depleted from chronic stress; chew your food thoroughly; eat meals at regular intervals combining quality fats, proteins and carbohydrates at each meal; eat within an hour of rising; green drinks and vegetable juicing; healthy fats (nuts, seeds, avocado, olive oil, sesame oil, coconut oil); herbal teas (chamomile, passion flower, valerian, licorice root); organic and locally grown foods, cage-free and grass-fed when possible; raw foods – consume 50-75% of your foods in their raw state, and consider sea vegetables such as kelp and wakame (seaweed salad).

R℥ Anti-Aging

Carrots, high in antioxidants and with an alkaline pH, give us healthy skin and protect against acne and aging. Increase raw food and fiber intake: vegetables, fruits, nuts, seeds, grains and include quality protein in diet (especially wild fish), with plenty of broccoli, cabbage, and cauliflower. Avoid processed foods. Use garlic, onions, shiitake mushrooms and pearl barley: these lessen free radical damage. Cut back on salt, avoid saturated fats, caffeine, red meat, white flour, white sugar, tap water. Exercise! Relax! Breathe deeply!

R℞ *Allergies, Seasonal*

20% of Americans suffer from allergies. Beware of drugstore remedies as they mask symptoms and often cause drowsiness – or worse side effects than the allergy itself. If you are allergic to ragweed don't eat cantaloupe (contains the same proteins). Aim for a plant-based diet as animal fats produce leukotrienes associated with allergies. If you are mucousy, consider a 3-5 day cleanse with celery juice, fresh fruits and vegetables (cabbage, onions, garlic) and plenty of pure water. Pollen counts are generally highest between 5am-10am, keep this is in mind for outdoor activities. Acupressure and acupuncture have been shown to be successful in relieving allergy symptoms. And of course, avoid smoking!

R℞ *Alzheimer's Disease*

Eat a well-balanced diet of natural foods. Red cabbage, with more phytonutrients than white cabbage, is a safeguard against Alzheimer's disease. Increase foods with vitamins A, E and the cartenoids; vitamin E can slow the advancement up to 25%. Investigate a vitamin B12 deficiency. Omega-3s: as the primary building block for brain tissue, they help you stay focused, supply oxygen to the brain, protect brain cell membranes, and decrease your chances of dementia, Alzheimer's, stroke, and other brain illnesses later in life.

Rx: Anxiety Attack

When experiencing a panic attack the fear is so great that one loses all sense of reality; some feel as though they might die. (Know that night anxiety and heart palpitations are common during menopause.) Avoid alcohol, caffeine, nicotine as they deplete B vitamins, natural sedatives for your body. Stay away from sugar, artificial sweeteners, fast food, MSG, fried food, cola beverages. Regular exercise reduces symptoms; yoga, and deep, slow, regular breathing will let your brain know that everything is ok. Eat foods rich in B vitamins: raw nuts and beans, and calcium: leafy greens, raw almonds and sesame seeds.

Rx: Arthritis

Arthritis can be reversible, and curable with proper diet and lifestyle changes. Eat more sulfuric foods: asparagus, eggs, garlic and onions (sulfur repairs bone, cartilage and connective tissue and aids in the absorption of calcium). Fresh leafy green vegetables with their vitamin K, non-acidic fresh fruits (especially cherries: eat 20/day), whole grains, oatmeal, brown rice, fish, soybean products and avocados will benefit. Avoid dairy, red meat, coffee and sugar. Avoid the nightshade vegetables: eggplant, peppers tomatoes, white potatoes – these contain solanine which interferes with enzymes in the muscles and may cause pain and discomfort. Alfalfa and kelp contain all minerals essential for bone formation. Ginger, a powerful antioxidant with anti-inflammatory effects, will help with pain and soreness; tumeric also (600 mg daily). Omega-3 essential fatty acids may alleviate symptoms of rheumatoid arthritis.

Rx: Asthma

First, stay hydrated. A significant portion of water loss (about a pint each day) experienced by the body each day is through respiration – a bit of water vapor is exhaled with each breath. Your body attempts to reduce water loss during respiration by constricting your bronchial tubes through the creation of histamines. The histamines constrict breathing, making it more physically difficult. The underlying cause of asthma may often simply be dehydration. So instead of prescribing water to solve the underlying water shortage and end the body's creation of histamines, doctors may prescribe anti-histamine drugs that force the bronchial tubes to relax and ease airflow. This promotes further dehydration, leaving the patient in a more severe state of water loss. High consumption of apples may protect against asthma; avoid processed foods and salt. Boswellia has been found to inhibit the formation of compounds called leukotrienes, which cause narrowing of airways. To calm asthma, honey is beneficial, mix a teaspoon into a glass of pure water and drink 3x/day. Ginger also, grate 1inch ginger root with 2 minced garlic cloves and boil as tea.

Rx: Bladder, Urinary Tract Infections

Nearly 85% of urinary tract infections are caused by *e coli* bacteria found in the intestines. Infections thrive in an environment of surplus acid-forming foods: avoid refined sugar, concentrated sweeteners. Cucumber juice treats kidney and bladder infections as it contains erepsis, a digestive enzyme that breaks down protein and cleanses the intestines. Eat 6oz whole cucumber, or 1 cup juice each day. Also incorporate: full fat whole yogurt (Greek or Fage brand), colloidal silver, garlic, Vitamin C (4-5,000 mg). No caffeine, orange juice, carbonated beverages, refined or processed foods. Use chlorophyll, aduki beans, celery, lemon, cranberry, blueberry, parsley, flax seed, Omega 3s and almonds.

Rx: Brain Power

Go for lean proteins, like fish, white meat, or eggs; protein helps your body manufacture two chemicals made from tyrosine: norepinephrine and dopamine which enable the synthesis of neurotransmitters and boost mental alertness. Healthy fats: essential fatty acids, or omega-3 fatty acids, your brain needs these to function optimally: wild salmon, walnuts, olive oil, avocados, and flax seed are great sources. Flax is also the best source of alphalinoleic, a healthy fat that enhances the performance of the cerebral cortex, where your brain processes sensory information. B vitamins, like vitamins B6, B12 and folic acid, are still proven to help your memory, focus, and overall brain health and power (folic acid helps produce red blood cells and improve your sense of wellbeing and mental clarity). Brown rice and quinoa are a great source of B vitamins, as are broccoli, parsley, cauliflower and brussels sprouts. Leafy green vegetables like kale, spinach, and Swiss chard, pack in high amounts of folic acid and vitamin K, which also help your brain focus and fight off memory disorders, like dementia.

R℘: Cancer prevention

Include a variety of grains, nuts, seeds and unpolished brown rice in your diet. Eat plenty of cruciferous vegetables: broccoli, Brussels sprouts, cauliflower, and spinach, and the deep yellow orange vegetables such as carrots, pumpkin, squash and yams; these reduce the risk of cancer. Cabbage, high in phytonutrients, lowers our risk of cancer in the lungs, prostate, colon, breasts, ovaries and bladder, and its phytochemicals can protect against bowel cancer. Green plants, high in chlorophyll, fight cancer. Berries protect DNA from damage; tart cherries also. The lycopene in tomatoes protects cells from cervical, lung, stomach and prostate cancers. Eat 7-10 servings of fresh fruits and vegetables each day. Green tea contains cancer-fighting properties, and curcumin, found in tumeric, may inhibit the rapid division of cancer cells. Eat 10 raw almonds every day; their laetrile has anti-cancer properties.

R℘ Candida, Yeast Infections

A healthy colon contains no more than 15 percent unhealthy bacteria and at least 85 percent healthy bacteria; the typical American has the opposite ratio. Candida albicans is a bacteria that thrives on sugar and causes yeast and other infections in the body. Limit the amount of soda, candy and other sweets to keep candida under control. Also, because complex carbohydrates are broken down into simple sugars by the body, do not consume excess amounts of breads, pastas, potatoes and rice. Probiotics, known as "friendly flora," include a group of bacterium that live in the digestive tract and help facilitate digestion, manufacture certain nutrients and even help keep unhealthy bacteria under control. The main probiotics include Lactobacillus acidophilus and Bifidobacterium bifidus, and are found in natural (Greek) yogurt, miso, tofu and sauerkraut. These powerful probiotics consume candida (yeast), fungi and other disease-causing bacteria such as E coli and salmonella. An effective probiotic should have at least a 10 billion bacterial count. Some women have found prompt relief from yeast infections by inserting a clove of garlic (without skin but intact) into the vagina for 12-24 hours. Others have had success dipping a tampon into a solution of one part tea tree oil, three parts water and inserting for 24 hours.

R℟: High cholesterol

Cut back on red meat; eat more fish. Salmon, sardines and mackerel are excellent sources of omega-3 essential fatty acids, noted for their ability, like aspirin, to thin blood slightly to reduce the risk of clots. Soluble fiber in particular, can help in reducing serum cholesterol; it acts like a sponge to absorb cholesterol in the digestive tract. Good sources include dried beans, brown rice and barley, and fruits – especially apples (organic, with skin), blueberries and grapes. Slow-cooked oatmeal, not instant, and ¾ cup is perfect. A good quality olive oil is excellent for lowering cholesterol as are almonds and walnuts.

R℟: Circles Under Your Eyes

Dark circles under the eyes can be caused by anemia, which makes the skin look pale and the area around the eyes look darker; the most common cause is not getting enough iron. Eat foods such as red meats, green leafy vegetables, eggs, if you are iron deficient. You may need to eliminate caffeinated beverages from your diet; these stimulate your hormonal glands, causing fatigue and exhaustion if over-consumed, eventually resulting in adrenal exhaustion. Allergies can also cause dark circles.

R℟: Circulatory Problems

In the average adult body there are approximately 60,000 miles of blood vessels (can wrap around the Earth twice!); some are as thick as your finger and others are as thin as a hair. The blood vessels provide the transportation network that allows your blood to carry nutrients and oxygen to each of your cells; the network also allows your blood to remove waste products. When blood becomes too thick it is not able to flow through the body's small capillaries, causing circulatory problems. Eliminate sugar, animal protein and fatty foods from your diet. Avoid stimulants: coffee, cola, tobacco. Be sure to eat plenty of fiber; this helps lower cholesterol. Eat bananas, brown rice, endive, garlic, spinach, pears, peas, onions and lima beans. Exercise regularly!

Rχ: Feeling congested/stuffed up? Cold and Upper Respiratory

Green and red peppers: Vitamin C, a natural antihistamine. Carrots' beta-carotene is converted to Vitamin A, helps boost immunity and keeps the respiratory system working optimally. It also is a powerful antioxidant. Through much experimentation we have found the Elderberry and Zinc lozenges to be an effective way to divert the onset of a cold. If the cold has taken hold, to clear sinuses, put the Neti Pot to use!

Rχ: Constipation or Diarrhea

Chew your food! Digestion begins in the mouth; chewing breaks down the food and releases digestive enzymes that allow food to be more easily absorbed. Eat foods with soluble fiber: oatmeal, sweet potatoes, carrots, beets, squash, rice cereals. Cabbage, with its fiber, Vitamin C, calcium, fiber and manganese will assist with cleansing the colon and provide healthy bacteria for healing. Pay attention to your stools: if you notice blood or mucus and this continues, consult your doctor. If the stools are flattened or ribbon-like it is usually a sign of an obstruction, possibly a polyp that narrows the pathway. Large, messy stools are a sign of malabsorption of nutrients, leads to nutritional deficiencies; you may have an intolerance or allergy; dairy, gluten and soy are common allergies. Abnormally fatty stools signal pancreas issues – inflammation of the pancreas can lead to diabetes. Extremely foul smelling stools may mean you have a deficiency of "friendly bacteria" in your intestines, a diet too high in red meat, protein or candida yeast overgrowth. With greenish stools, cut down on sugar. If you are a vegetarian who doesn't consume a lot of sugar, this may mean you need more whole grains in your diet. Pale, grayish stools can be a sign of liver or gallbladder problems. Dark brown stools can be the result of too much salt in the diet. Black, tar-like stools may mean you have bleeding in your upper digestive tract.

R*χ* Diabetes, Type II

See above Circulatory entry. With Type II Diabetes, (affecting 90-95% of those with diabetes) the pancreas does not produce enough insulin to fuel the cells, or the cells have become resistant to the insulin in the bloodstream. This is potentially devastating as your network of blood vessels can slowly become clogged up, destroying the transportation system that your blood relies on to nourish and cleanse your cells. Left unchecked, diabetes can result in complete blockages to your circulatory system, paving the way to every known health challenge, the most common being kidney and heart disease, neurological disease, vision loss, amputation due to impaired blood circulation and sexual dysfunction. Many with Type II Diabetes are completely unaware of it; often they cannot perceive sweet flavors. Eat a low-fat, high fiber diet based on raw fruits and vegetables and fresh juices. Fiber helps reduce blood sugar surges, as does spirulina. Use legumes for protein, avoid saturated fats. Consistent intake of magnesium-rich foods can significantly lower your risk of developing diabetes. These include: brown rice, raw almonds, spinach, Swiss chard, lima beans, avocado, raw hazelnuts, okra and black-eyed peas. Talk to a health professional about the right approach to exercise.

R℥: Dry Skin

The skin is our largest organ; moisture is the water inside the skin cells that comes through the bloodstream. A balance of oil and moisture is crucial for healthy skin; oil is secreted though the sebaceous glands, lubricating the skin's surface. Vitamin A and B deficiencies can contribute to dry skin. Aloe vera can soothe and heal skin; it sloughs dead skin cells. Aim for a diet of vegetables, fruits, grains, raw seeds and nuts, and foods that are high in sulfur like garlic, onions, eggs and asparagus. Drink at least 2 quarts of water daily for skin hydration. No soft drinks, sugar, junk foods and no smoking!

R℘: *Eczema*

There are a number of underlying causes that can lead to eczema: low levels of hydrochloric acid in the stomach, leaky gut, candidiasis, food or other allergies. Include brown rice and millet in your diet; avoid eggs, peanuts, all soy, wheat (avoid all gluten) and dairy, as well as processed foods and sugar. EFAs (essential fatty acids) like krill and salmon oil will promote lubrication of the skin; kelp (1,000mg per day) will heal tissues; zinc (100mg daily) will aid healing and promote immune function. For external treatment apply raw honey, rub with fresh slices of papaya; the juice of daikon radish or raw organic potato can also be applied as a wash.

R℘: *Increase your energy*

With half of our population sleep deprived, most people feel tired; some don't have energy for the events of daily life. While it's practical and easy to turn to coffee, colas, sugar and other substances, these ultimately lead to greater energy reduction and larger challenges. Natural energizers have the advantage of not exhausting the body; they support vs. deplete. First, aim for adequate sleep! Immune response will increase and blood pressure will lower. Winter squashes and root vegetables are known for their influence on the spleen-pancreas and the stomach, and for improving energy and circulation, and are great source of natural sugars, beta-carotene and carbohydrates – great choice for diabetics and for those with digestive problems. Start with a protein drink in the morning, reduce or eliminate dairy. Aim for 65% good carbs from fresh vegetables, fruits, legumes and grains; 25% protein from nuts, seeds, yogurt, clean meats; 10% quality fats from olive oil, nuts. Stretching and deep breathing do wonders for energy, as does yoga or a brisk walk. Ginseng and B complex vitamins will provide healthy boost!

Rχ: Fibroids

20-30% of all women develop fibroid tumors, usually late 30s-early 40s, and African-American women are 3x more likely to have fibroids than other women. Obesity increases risk. Avoid coffee and caffeinated beverages, sugary and salty foods. Aim for a 60% fresh food mostly vegetarian diet with whole grains like brown rice, sprouts, raw nuts and seeds, wild seafoods, organic poultry. Increase cabbage, broccoli, cauliflower Brussels sprouts and high fiber foods like organic apples (with skin). Add cucumber and carrot juice, and plenty of water. Tumeric, dandelion and evening primrose oil are recommended, as is acupuncture.

Rχ: Food Allergies

Most food and chemical reactions are considered *sensitivities*. A food sensitivity sounds benign, but in fact in can be a contributing factor to many disease conditions, including asthma, headaches, behavioral issues, digestive problems, autism, ear infections, and more. Allergy refers to the immune system's hypersensitivity to an offending substance whereby specific antibodies become elevated due to an antigen. It is the immune system's reaction to a substance that other people find harmless.

Allergic reactions are classified into two categories, immediate and delayed (up to 72 hours), and can range from mild to severe (can cause anaphylactic shock). The most common food allergies include milk and milk products, gluten, soy, nuts especially peanuts, soy, eggs and shellfish. Eliminating milk products can help diminish the symptoms of other allergies, (and don't worry about the calcium – just eat plenty of leafy greens, like the cows do). Enhancing the bacteria in your gut may also be helpful (see Candida posting). Consuming naturally fermented vegetables (no vinegar) like sauerkraut, pickles and unpasteurized miso will provide probiotic elements. Try eating two tablespoons of sauerkraut[13] per day.

Rχ: Gout

Gout is one of more than one hundred manifestations of arthritis. It occurs when levels of uric acid are abnormally elevated causing severe attacks of pain, swelling, redness, and inflammation. Needle shaped uric acid crystals stab their way into joints rendering lightning bolts of pain. When an attack occurs, eat only raw fruits and vegetables for two weeks, and drink cherry juice and celery juice diluted with pure water. Strawberries and blueberries will neutralize uric acid. Other safe foods during an

---

[1] Natural sauerkraut recipe: Cut a small cabbage in quarters, top to bottom, and cut out the core. Slice the quarters into thin strips, and spread them out. Sprinkle strips with sea salt, Place in a porcelain crock or glass pot. Put a plate on top with some weights, to press down. Place in a dark and cool spot. Next day, take a look: enough water should have been released to cover the cabbage. If not, add some warm water, with one teaspoon of sea salt per cup, stir well, and pour enough to cover the cabbage by one inch. Let sit about a week; remove anything on top of the water. Pour into a clean glass jar with the water and keep covered in the fridge. (recipe from Annemarie Colbin, Ph.D.)

episode are rice, millet, starchy vegetables, green vegetables, corn, seeds and grains. Foods to avoid are: meat of any kind, sardines, scallops, shellfish, mushrooms, mussels, peanuts, mackerel, asparagus, alcohol beverages, and diet soda. Limit your intake of caffeine, cauliflower, dried beans and lentils, oatmeal, peas, spinach and yeast products.[14]

R℞ Hangover

Limeade stimulates the liver, flushes out toxins and stabilizes blood sugar. Lime contains antioxidant, anti-carcinogenic, antibiotic and detoxifying flavonoids that alleviate nausea, congestion, flush out the excretory system, and help the kidneys to purge toxic substances from the body. Slowly drinking an 8 ounce glass of water with 1 teaspoon of sugar and 2 teaspoons of freshly squeezed lime juice will help to offset the damage that you did the night before. The chlorophyll in *wheatgrass*, a natural detoxifier, offers so many valuable body-enhancing benefits, including water/blood cleansing effects and powerful antioxidant capabilities that recharge the cells; it is also believed to alleviate high blood pressure, drain the lymphatic system, restore energy. Fresh *cabbage* contains large amounts of vitamin C as well as the anti-inflammatory amino acid glutamine and is used to treat acute inflammation, offer relief for headaches and help aid the metabolic process of alcohol assimilation. *Ginger root*, famous for alleviating motion sickness, indigestion and unsettled stomachs; brewing fresh ginger root in boiling water for at least 20 minutes releases a spicy, flavorful tea that can effectively flush your system when sipping continually through-out the day.

Rχ: Heart Health

Heart disease is the biggest killer in the US (and women are 50% more at risk then men), and it is 100% preventable with diet and lifestyle changes! Keep your arteries clear and your blood slippery! Avoid overly rich foods, all saturated fats as well as sugar, coffee, late-night eating. Take good quality B vitamins! Folic acid lowers cardiovascular risk 45% in women. Use gluten-free, whole grains like brown rice, steel cut oatmeal. Potassium-rich foods: spinach, chard, bananas, sea greens, papaya, broccoli, all mushrooms, especially reishi. Silicon foods such as cucumber, celery improve calcium metabolism and strengthen nerve and heart tissue. Green foods. Also apples, cabbage, chia seed, apple cider vinegar and blue-green algae (1 t vinegar 3x daily and 1.5 g wild blue-green algae 1-3x daily). Garlic (1200mg daily) main-tains aortic elasticity as does ginger. CoQ10 strengethens the heart muscle and helps it work more effectively.

Rχ: Heartburn, GERD

When it comes to digestion, often what is thought to be an overly acidic condition can, in fact, be *weak* stomach acid in need of stronger acid to properly digest foods. The best way to test this is to swallow a teaspoon of vinegar with your meal and see wheth-er you feel better or worse. The vinegar will usually halt the pain normally felt after eating, indicating stomach acid production is lacking. To encourage production of healthy stomach acid, drink fresh vegetable juices each day—especially celery and cabbage juices. Aloe vera juice aids healing of the intestinal tract and chamomile tea can relieve esophageal irritation. With the first signs of heartburn, drink a glass of water: hydration is key. Eat plenty of raw vegetables, eat slowly, chewing your food very well. Fresh papaya and pineapple will aid digestion. No carbonated beverages, processed foods, sugar or highly spiced foods.

Rx: High Blood Pressure

Most healthy adults need 1,500-2,400 milligrams (mg) of sodium a day. If you have high blood pressure, are older than 50, are black, or have heart disease, kidney disease or diabetes, you may be more sensitive to sodium: aim for less than 1,500mg a day (1 level teaspoon of salt has 2,300mg). Just a modest reduction in sodium can reduce blood pressure. Avoid processed foods, frozen dinners; use kelp, dulse, herbs and spices to add more flavor to your foods. In the many cases, high blood pressure means you simply need more water, more living nutrients (such as raw living plant juices), more omega-3 fatty acids and a sharp reduction in the consumption of animal products. (also see Circulation entry)

R℞: Hypoglycemia (low blood sugar)

More and more people today have hypoglycemia due to poor dietary habits, including eating large quantities of carbohydrates, sugars, alcohol, caffeine and soft drinks – high levels of stress also contribute. Milk allergy is common with this disorder. To manage hypoglycemia, remove all alcohol, packaged, canned, refined and processed foods, salt, sugar (use stevia to sweeten foods), saturated fats, soft drinks, white flour and all foods with artificial colors or preservatives. Aim for a high-fiber diet plentiful in raw vegetables, especially broccoli, carrots and spinach. Eat beans and brown rice, oats, lentils, apples, avocados and lemons. Maintain a regular exercise program and consider fasting one day a month, using only fresh vegetable juices.

R℞: Inflammation

Evaluating and choosing the best natural anti-inflammatory depends on the specific condition, but the primary arsenal of herbal remedies includes ginger, turmeric, boswellia, bromelain, glucosamine sulfate, omega-3 essential fats, slippery elm, fenugreek, and devil's claw root. Curcumin is the primary active anti-inflammatory component of turmeric; it contains antioxidant, antiviral, and antifungal properties. Like ginger, it inhibits the enzymes and prostaglandins that play a role in inflammation. Eating a diet rich in wild fish, fresh fruits and vegetables, nuts, and seeds is the best way to prevent inflammatory conditions. Blueberries and cranberries provide polyphenolic protection against sight-damaging inflammation and oxidative stress.

Cherries (the tarter the better) are another inflammation-fighting food. Limit or eliminate red meat, alcohol, hydrogenated fats, refined sugars, and flours.[15]

Rχ: Kidney/Bladder Infection

Nearly 85% of urinary tract infections are caused by e-coli bacteria found in the intestines. Infections thrive in an environment of surplus acid-forming foods: avoid refined sugar, concentrated sweeteners. Cucumber juice treats kidney and bladder infections as it contains erepsis, a digestive enzyme that breaks down protein and cleanses the intestines. Eat 6 oz whole cucumber, or 1 cup juice each day. Also incorporate: full fat whole yogurt (Greek or FAGE), colloidal silver, garlic, Vitamin C (4-5,000 mg). No caffeine, orange juice, carbonated beverages, refined or processed foods. Use chlorophyll, aduki beans, celery, lemon, cranberry, blueberry, parsley, flax seed, Omega 3s and almonds.

Rχ: Kidney Stones

Over 10x more common now than at the beginning of the 20th century, kidney stones are the accumulation of mineral salts that become lodged in the urinary tract. They can be extremely painful, with pain radiating to the upper back to lower groin, chills and fever. About 10% of Americans develop kidney stones, primarily Southern white men aged 30-50. There are four types of kidney stones: calcium, uric acid, struvite and cystine stones and 80% are calcium oxalate stones whereby the excess calcium in the system forms a stone. Consumption of refined carbohy-drates, especially sugar, can precipitate this, as does dehydration. Drink 3 quarts of water daily; fresh lemon in warm water upon waking is a preventative measure. Increase vitamin A foods: carrots, pumpkin, sweet potato, alfalfa, apricots, cantaloupes. Minimize animal protein, salt, refined sugar and soft drinks. Stay active!

Rx: Liver Support

Start your morning with fresh lemon juice in water; this helps flush and decongest the liver. Eat beets or drink beet and vegetable juice regularly, as well as chlorophyll drinks and other green drinks. High quality protein foods are necessary to restore and sustain the liver. Free-range eggs, fish, raw nuts and seeds and whole grains are beneficial. Nutritional antioxidants such as vitamin E, zinc and selenium are essential for protecting the liver from free radical damage. A minimum of 2 quarts of pure water daily. Milk thistle, dandelion or burdock can be taken two to three times daily. Dandelion root is considered ideal because it is completely non-toxic and gently restores liver function; it enhances the flow of bile and supports the kidneys during cleansing and detoxification of the liver and bowels.

R℞ *Macular Degeneration*

Macular degeneration is the leading cause of blindness in the US affecting over 13 million over 60 years old. Vision becomes blurried and distorted; glasses do not help. It is associated with smokers, UV sunlight, low carotene and can be reversed with a robust nutritional therapy. A diet enriched in EPA and DHA (docosahexaenoic acid, an omega-3 fatty acid) can ameliorate the progression of retinal lesions. The carotenoid lutein—found in many vegetables including carrots, kale, collard greens, mangos, tomatoes, and parsley—may prevent macular degeneration as well as cataracts; dark greens can cut risk up to 50%. Zinc rich foods: all sea foods and sea vegetables, beans, pumpkin seeds.[16]

R℞ *Nail Health*

Nail abnormalities can reveal an underlying disorder. Nails that peel or break easily show inadequate hydrochloric acid and protein. Vertical ridges indicate poor nutrient absorption or iron deficiency, or a kidney disorder. Horizontal ridges can manifest as a result of severe stress To strengthen nails, soak in warm olive oil or cider vinegar 10-20 minutes each day. Artificial nails destroy the underlying nail and contribute to infection.

R℞ *Night Vision?*

Carrots! The body converts the carrot's beta-carotene into Vitamin A, which allows us to see in dim light and enhances overall vision health. Carrots can prevent macular degeneration (see entry), a medical condition found predominantly in the elderly whereby the macula area of the retina, the center of the inner lining of the eye, thins, atrophies, and in some cases, bleeds. The result is a loss of central vision: the inability to see fine details, read or recognize faces.

R℞ Oily Skin

Oily skin is usually genetic but can be affected by diet, hormone levels and cosmetics. It occurs when the oil-secreting glands produce more oil than is needed for lubrication of the skin; the pores become clogged and blemishes can appear. As with dry skin, aloe vera applied topically has excellent healing properties. Drink plenty of water to flush out toxins. Reduce the fat in your diet – no fried foods, watch for hydrogenated oils in all packaged foods – use olive oil only. No soft drinks, avoid sugar and junk food. Keep your skin clean, avoiding harsh cleansers that contain alcohol. Try mixing equal parts of lemon juice and water, pat on face, allow to dry, rinse with warm then cool water.

R℞ Osteoporosis

Meaning "porous bones," this is a progressive disease where the bones become weaker and weaker; osteoporosis affects many more women than men – half of all women 45-75 have signs (women of African descent are less likely to be affected). For all, after age 30 bones begin to weaken, and for women this accelerates with menopause due to the loss of estrogen which causes an increase in loss of bone minerals. Lack of regular exercise speeds the loss of bone mass, as do smoking and caffeine. Eat foods that are high in calcium-magnesium-potassium foods rich in vitamin D, such as broccoli, dandelion greens, sprouts, dark leafy greens, kelp, oysters, salmon, sardines (with bones). Include garlic and onions, organic eggs and yogurt (has 300 mg of calcium/cup). Include vitamin C foods, too: oranges, grapefruit, kiwis, fresh pineapple juice.

R℞: PMS

Diet is an important contributing factor in overcoming PMS; the anxiety, abdominal bloating, acne, fatigue and other imbalances occurring prior to the period are due to uneven hormonal fluctuations. PMS has also been linked to food allergies, malabsorption of nutrients and hypoglycemia. Eat less dairy, avoid caffeine, no alcohol or sugar in the week leading up to symptoms. Regular exercise to oxygenate blood, aiding nutrient absorption and elimination of toxins. No smoking! Plenty of fresh fruits and vegetables; protein snacks between meals. Tons of water, no salt, no caffeine, processed or junk foods. Acupuncture and meditation can be helpful. Consider having you thyroid checked; many suffering from PMS also have thyroid dysfunction.

R℞: Rosacea

When groups of capillaries close to the skin's surface become dilated, this flushing of the face and cheeks is caused by swelling of the blood vessels. Rosacea is most common in fair-skinned women, aged 30-50 and can be aggravated by alcohol, humidity, stress, vitamin deficiency and spicy foods. There is no known cure, however a diet rich in raw vegetables and organic grains is advised. Avoid saturated fats as they promote inflammation. Keep a food journal to see which foods may be exacerbating the rosacea, investigate food allergies.

R℣: S.A.D. (Seasonal Affective Disorder)

Women are more likely than men to experience SAD; in the winter months many become depressed, lose energy, experience anxiety attacks and weight gain. Eating complex carbohydrates, salmon and turkey raises the level of tryptophan in the brain, which triggers serotonin production and has a calming effect. Avoid wheat; gluten has been linked to depressive disorders. Avoid aspartame and diet sodas; this sweetener blocks the formation of serotonin. Avoid fried and junk foods, sugar, alcohol and caffeine. Keep your mind actively engaged in constructive thinking. Light therapy is worth considering, as is the thyroid, which may be underactive.

R℣: Sinus Infections, congestion

Situated above the eyes, either side of the nose, behind the bridge and in the upper nose, and inside the cheekbones, sinuses are air-filled pockets connected to the nose and throat by passages designed to drain mucus away. In protecting the lungs from infection, the sinuses are the first line of defense. To avoid or manage infection, aim for a diet of 75% raw foods, fresh fruit and vegetable juices, plenty of hot liquids like soups and herb tea. Consider adding garlic, ginger, horseradish, cayenne for quick relief. Eliminate dairy (except yogurt) and sugar. Avoid over the counter decongestants: Neti Pot works wonders.

Rx: Ulcer

One of 10 Americans has ulcers! And approximately 10,000 die each year from ulcer complications. Smokers, big drinkers, eaters of rich or refined foods, as well as asprin-takers are prime candidates. Gastric or stomach ulcers occur in the upper stomach lining – pain is felt right after eating. Duodenal ulcers are felt several hours after eating. The most common, peptic ulcer is an erosion of the stomach lining, small intestine or esophagus. Most ulcers are caused by *H.pylori* bacteria, and a natural approach recreates intestinal balance. Drinking a cup of cabbage juice four times a day can heal stomach ulcers in just ten days (if time prevents juicing cabbage, purchase dehydrated, raw cabbage powder at natural food stores). The glutamine has proved to be a better ulcer cure than antacids. Eat small meals, chew well, easily digestible, fresh alkalizing foods: leafy greens, lightly steamed vegetables, whole grains and cultured foods like yogurt and kefir to promote friendly bacteria.[17]

Rx: Weight loss

By now, one out of 2 Americans is overweight! In children, one of 3 born after 2000 will become obese. About 300,000 die from issues contributing to obesity, and this is entirely preventable! Watch portion size, reduce fat to 15% of food intake (no "low fat" items, these are high in sugar, the same result). Slow down when eating, and don't eat in front of the tv or computer, or distract yourself in any way. Chew each bite 15 times, don't reload until the mouth is clean and enjoy the flavors, smelling and tasting. The cruciferous vegetables: cabbage, broccoli, kale, cauliflower, bok choy, are high in phytonutrients, which work to disarm free radicals before they damage DNA, cells, fat molecules such as cholesterol. Broccoli also contains more vitamin C than citrus, A, beta carotene, B vitamins, chlorophyll, fiber and powerful antioxidants – these all contribute to a sense of fullness and wellbeing. Go for a "quick exit" strategy with foods, where their vital nutrients are being absorbed and then they promptly leave the body. More fiber! 25g will keep things moving. A toxic buid-up may be responsible for weight gain; bitter greens will pull toxins and fat, bulk up on dandelion greens, arugula, watercress. Reduce your stress levels, move the body!

Grocery Lists

✂ Tear-out Grocery List - - - - - - - - - - - - - - - - -

☐ Water

Greens

☐ Spinach
☐ Collard Greens
☐ Kale
☐ Swiss Chard
☐ Watercress
☐ Dandelion Greens
☐ Mustard Greens
☐ Beet Greens

Veggies

☐ Broccoli
☐ Carrots, organic
☐ Celery, organic
☐ Bok Choy
☐ Rabe
☐ Cabbage, red or green
☐ Zucchini
☐ Garlic
☐ Onions
☐ Mushrooms

- ☐ Peppers, green, red, orange or yellow
- ☐ Eggplant
- ☐ Leeks
- ☐ Acorn Squash
- ☐ Turnips
- ☐ Parsnips
- ☐ Cauliflower

Grains

- ☐ Quinoa, red and white
- ☐ Millet
- ☐ Kasha
- ☐ Brown Rice
- ☐ Wild Rice
- ☐ Oatmeal
- ☐ Muesli
- ☐ Rice Pasta
- ☐ Sprouted Bread

Proteins

- ☐ Eggs, organic
- ☐ Red Meat, organic
- ☐ Chicken, organic
- ☐ Pork, organic
- ☐ Fish, wild
- ☐ Lentils
- ☐ Black beans
- ☐ Garbanzos
- ☐ Kidney beans
- ☐ Seaweed: nori
- ☐ Seaweed: wakame

Fats

- ☐ Olive oil
- ☐ Grape seed oil
- ☐ Coconut oil
- ☐ Almond Butter
- ☐ Peanut Butter
- ☐ Cashew Butter
- ☐ Avocado
- ☐ Sardines

Fruits

- ☐ Apples, organic
- ☐ Bananas
- ☐ Blueberries, fresh or frozen, organic
- ☐ Cherries
- ☐ Lemons
- ☐ Pears
- ☐ Peaches, organic – in season
- ☐ Nectarines, organic – in season

Snacks

- ☐ Almonds, raw
- ☐ Walnuts, raw
- ☐ Dried fruits
- ☐ Figs
- ☐ Apples, organic
- ☐ Yogurt
- ☐ 70% Cacao chocolate

Dairy

- ☐ Butter, unsalted
- ☐ Raw Milk
- ☐ Yogurt, Fage brand or Greek
- ☐ Almond Milk
- ☐ Rice Milk
- ☐ Oat Milk
- ☐ Hemp Milk
- ☐ Goat Cheese
- ☐ Sheep Cheese
- ☐ Try New Cheeses!

- -

Grocery Lists

✂ *Tear-out Grocery List* - - - - - - - - - - - - - - - - - -

☐ Water

Greens

☐ Spinach
☐ Collard Greens
☐ Kale
☐ Swiss Chard
☐ Watercress
☐ Dandelion Greens
☐ Mustard Greens
☐ Beet Greens

Veggies

☐ Broccoli
☐ Carrots, organic
☐ Celery, organic
☐ Bok Choy
☐ Rabe
☐ Cabbage, red or green
☐ Zucchini
☐ Garlic
☐ Onions
☐ Mushrooms

- ☐ Peppers, green, red, orange or yellow
- ☐ Eggplant
- ☐ Leeks
- ☐ Acorn Squash
- ☐ Turnips
- ☐ Parsnips
- ☐ Cauliflower

Grains

- ☐ Quinoa, red and white
- ☐ Millet
- ☐ Kasha
- ☐ Brown Rice
- ☐ Wild Rice
- ☐ Oatmeal
- ☐ Muesli
- ☐ Rice Pasta
- ☐ Sprouted Bread

Proteins

- ☐ Eggs, organic
- ☐ Red Meat, organic
- ☐ Chicken, organic
- ☐ Pork, organic
- ☐ Fish, wild
- ☐ Lentils
- ☐ Black beans
- ☐ Garbanzos
- ☐ Kidney beans
- ☐ Seaweed: nori
- ☐ Seaweed: wakame

Fats

- ☐ Olive oil
- ☐ Grape seed oil
- ☐ Coconut oil
- ☐ Almond Butter
- ☐ Peanut Butter
- ☐ Cashew Butter
- ☐ Avocado
- ☐ Sardines

Fruits

- ☐ Apples, organic
- ☐ Bananas
- ☐ Blueberries, fresh or frozen, organic
- ☐ Cherries
- ☐ Lemons
- ☐ Pears
- ☐ Peaches, organic – in season
- ☐ Nectarines, organic – in season

Snacks

- ☐ Almonds, raw
- ☐ Walnuts, raw
- ☐ Dried fruits
- ☐ Figs
- ☐ Apples, organic
- ☐ Yogurt
- ☐ 70% Cacao chocolate

Dairy

- ☐ Butter, unsalted
- ☐ Raw Milk
- ☐ Yogurt, Fage brand or Greek
- ☐ Almond Milk
- ☐ Rice Milk
- ☐ Oat Milk
- ☐ Hemp Milk
- ☐ Goat Cheese
- ☐ Sheep Cheese
- ☐ Try New Cheeses!

- -

Grocery Lists

✂ *Tear-out Grocery List* - - - - - - - - - - - - - - - - -

- ☐ Water

Greens

- ☐ Spinach
- ☐ Collard Greens
- ☐ Kale
- ☐ Swiss Chard
- ☐ Watercress
- ☐ Dandelion Greens
- ☐ Mustard Greens
- ☐ Beet Greens

Veggies

- ☐ Broccoli
- ☐ Carrots, organic
- ☐ Celery, organic
- ☐ Bok Choy
- ☐ Rabe
- ☐ Cabbage, red or green
- ☐ Zucchini
- ☐ Garlic
- ☐ Onions
- ☐ Mushrooms

- ☐ Peppers, green, red, orange or yellow
- ☐ Eggplant
- ☐ Leeks
- ☐ Acorn Squash
- ☐ Turnips
- ☐ Parsnips
- ☐ Cauliflower

Grains

- ☐ Quinoa, red and white
- ☐ Millet
- ☐ Kasha
- ☐ Brown Rice
- ☐ Wild Rice
- ☐ Oatmeal
- ☐ Muesli
- ☐ Rice Pasta
- ☐ Sprouted Bread

Proteins

- ☐ Eggs, organic
- ☐ Red Meat, organic
- ☐ Chicken, organic
- ☐ Pork, organic
- ☐ Fish, wild
- ☐ Lentils
- ☐ Black beans
- ☐ Garbanzos
- ☐ Kidney beans
- ☐ Seaweed: nori
- ☐ Seaweed: wakame

Fats

- ☐ Olive oil
- ☐ Grape seed oil
- ☐ Coconut oil
- ☐ Almond Butter
- ☐ Peanut Butter
- ☐ Cashew Butter
- ☐ Avocado
- ☐ Sardines

Fruits

- ☐ Apples, organic
- ☐ Bananas
- ☐ Blueberries, fresh or frozen, organic
- ☐ Cherries
- ☐ Lemons
- ☐ Pears
- ☐ Peaches, organic – in season
- ☐ Nectarines, organic – in season

Snacks

- ☐ Almonds, raw
- ☐ Walnuts, raw
- ☐ Dried fruits
- ☐ Figs
- ☐ Apples, organic
- ☐ Yogurt
- ☐ 70% Cacao chocolate

Dairy

- ☐ Butter, unsalted
- ☐ Raw Milk
- ☐ Yogurt, Fage brand or Greek
- ☐ Almond Milk
- ☐ Rice Milk
- ☐ Oat Milk
- ☐ Hemp Milk
- ☐ Goat Cheese
- ☐ Sheep Cheese
- ☐ Try New Cheeses!

- -

Footnotes and References

1 **Protein Chapter References**

Healing with Whole Foods, by Paul Pitchford, pages 506-511

Food and Healing, by Annemarie Colbin, pages 169-71

Integrative Nutrition, by Joshua Rosenthal, pages 177-181

The Self-Healing Cookbook, by Kristina Turner, pages 76-77

Energetics of Food, by Steve Gagné, pages 229-238

Prescription for Nutritional Healing, Phyllis A. Balch. page 4

Healthy Healing, Linda Page, page 142

2 **Vegetable Chapter References**

Energetics of Food, by Steve Gagné, pages 197-198

The Self-Healing Cookbook, by Kristina Turner, pages 68 and 70

Healing with Whole Foods, by Paul Pitchford, page 329

Integrative Nutrition, by Joshua Rosenthal, pages 115-116

Greens Glorious Greens, by Johnna Albi and Catherine Walthers

Healthy Healing, by Linda Page, p126

[3]   Ludger Schmiech, Daisuke Uemura and Thomas Hofmann, *Journal of Agricultural and Food Chemistry,* 2008.

[4]   Worthington , Virginia . Nutritional Quality of Organic Versus Conventional Fruits, Vegetables, and Grains. *The Journal of Alternative and Complementary Medicine.* Vol. 7, 2. 2001.

[5]   Lorette C. Luzajic. Source: http://gremolata.com/soytrouble.htm

http://www.westonaprice.org/soy/darkside.html and Dianne Gregg, *The Hidden Dangers of Soy,* www.hiddensoy.com

[6]   Whole Grains Council/Oldways Preservation Trust www.oldwayspt.org

[7]   *Fat and Blood,* BiblioBazaar, LLC, 2007. Mitchell, S.W., (pp. 119-154).

The Miracle of Milk- How to Use the Milk Diet Scientifically at Home, *Read Books,* 2008. McFadden, B.

[8]   see http://www.realmilk.com/where1.html

[9]   see http://milk.procon.org/view.answers.php?questionID= 000808

[10]   Chanjirakul, K., Wang, S.Y., Wang, C.Y., Siriphanich, J. 2007. Natural volatile treatments increase free radical scavenging capacity of strawberries and blackberries. *Journal of the Science of Food and Agriculture.* 87:1463-1472.

11 **Fruits Chart References:**

www.botanical.com/products/learn/oilprofile/
pomegranate_seed.html

www.webmd.com/prostate-cancer/news/20060705/
pomegranate-slows-prostate-cancer

Pomegranate Seed Oil Causes Breast Cancer Cells to Self-Destruct, *Technion - Israel Institute ofTechnology.*

info@ats.org

Exotic Antioxidant Superfruits - Pomegranate: Review of current research. 2007/03/30 - By Dr. Paul Gross

12 Institute for Integrative Nutrition, curriculum

13 Natural sauerkraut recipe: Cut a small cabbage in quarters, top to bottom, and cut out the core. Slice the quarters into thin strips, and spread them out. Sprinkle strips with sea salt. Place in a porcelain crock or glass pot. Put a plate on top with some weights, to press down. Place in a dark and cool spot. Next day, take a look: enough water should have been released to cover the cabbage. If not, add some warm water, with one teaspoon of sea salt per cup, stir well, and pour enough to cover the cabbage by one inch. Let sit about a week; remove anything on top of the water. Pour into a clean glass jar with the water and keep covered in the fridge. (recipe from Annemarie Colbin, Ph.D., http://community.wddty.com/blogs/fooddoctor/archive/2008/05/12/Anti_2D00_allergy-foods.aspx)

[14] *Natural News,* Deanna Dean. Monday, January 11, 2010. http://www.NaturalNews.com/027910_gout_natural_remedi es.html

[15] Lucretia Schanfarber *alive* #262, August 2004

[16] Tuo J, Ross RJ, Herzlich AA, Shen D, Ding X, Zhou M, Coon SL, Hussein N, Salem Jr N, Chan C-C: A high omega-3 fatty acid diet reduces retinal lesions in a murine model of macular degeneration. *American Journal of Pathology,* 2009 175: 799-807.

[17] *Herbs for Health and Healing* by Kathi Keville. 1998.

References

Albi, Johanna & Walthers, *Catherine. Greens, Gorious Greens!* 1996.

Balch, Phyllis A. *Prescription for Nutritional Healing.* 2000.

Bittman, Mark. *Food Matters.* 2009.

Colbin, Annemarie. *Food and Healing.* 1986.

D'Adamo, Peter J. and Whitney, Catherine. *Eat Right For Your Type.* 1996.

Gagné, Steve. *Energetics of Food.* Healing Arts Press. 2008.

Gittleman, Ann Louise. *Your Body Knows Best.* 1997.

Nestle, Marion. *What to Eat.* 2006

Page, Linda. *Healthy Healing.* 2004.

Pitchford, Paul. *Healing with Whole Foods.* 2002.

Pollan, Michael. *In Defense of Food.* 2008.

Rose, Natalia. *The Raw Food Detox Diet.* 2005.

Rosenthal, Joshua. *Integrative Nutrition.* 2006.

Turner, Kristina. *The Self-Healing Cookbook.* Earthtones Press, 2002.

Willett, Walter C., M.D. *Eat, Drink, and Be Healthy.* President and Fellows of Harvard College, 2001.

Index

Note: Main page references are printed in **boldface**; references to items in charts and table are followed by a "**t.**"

Biographies

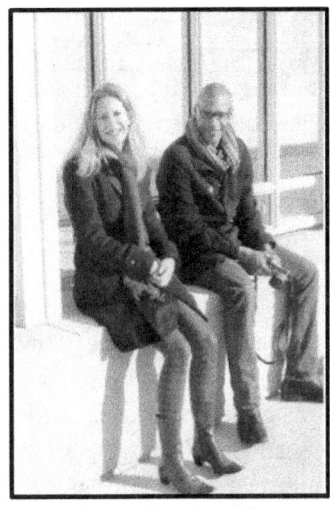

Photo: Claire Laveglia

Martin E. Rollins is a Holistic Health Counselor who was raised in Detroit, MI. In school studying Philosophy in 2005 he found himself captivated by the effects of Hurricane Katrina. It was the exposure – the vastness – of the cultural habits of the poor that clearly precipitated many deaths. His observations went beyond the physical devastation and confused government involvement, further into diet and, in particular, mindset. Rollins had the realization that the isolation of those in New Orleans was reminiscent of what he witnessed growing up in Detroit. He realized his own awareness came not only from his culture but his accountability for his choices.

Meanwhile, at his day job at the American Dietetic Association (creators of the "Healthy Eating" Pyramid) he found himself listening to the food-cultural 'disconnects' of consumers and decided in 2006 to begin a more formal training in holistic nutrition. He graduated from New York's Institute for Integrative Nutrition in 2007 and was awarded a certificate for those studies through Columbia University's Teachers College. He is a member of the American Association of Drugless Practitioners. Rollins lives in Chicago where he and co-author Joelle Rabion launched **rr holistic health** (www.rrholistichealth.com) and **Good Food, Better Life** (www.goodfoodbetterlife.com) in 2008. When he witnessed the improvement in his mother's life after her 40-lb weight loss, Rollins investigated the methodology and then became trained as a Sadkhin Practitioner, where he currently facilitates the healing of individuals using an organ detoxification technique.

~

Joelle Rabion was raised bi-culturally with a French father and American mother, allowing first hand experience with "The French Paradox". Her passion for the healing power of food is far-reaching, and having completed the program at the Institute for Integrative Nutrition with Rollins in 2007, as a holistic health counselor and meal consultant she actively helps others improve the quality of their lives. Rabion speaks and presents workshops on a wide variety of health topics, and also provides custom formulations for food and beverages in the nutrition, health and functional food markets, including product development and marketing services. Rabion's previous publications include: "Art in Chicago" and "Photography in Chicago", *Sweet Home Chicago*, Chicago Review Press, 1992.

Rollins and Rabion have expanded their counseling practice beyond the Chicago region throughout the US where they work with clients and provide corporate consultation on preventive medicine, healing through whole foods, and, of course, accountability.